THE SEVEN
ARCHETYPAL
STONES

"Nicholas Pearson's book *The Seven Archetypal Stones* is well researched and beautifully written, offering new insights, meditations, and practices for seven of the most fascinating stones in history. It is refreshing to see a new generation of crystal authors like Nicholas Pearson."

KATRINA RAPHAELL,
AUTHOR OF THE CRYSTAL TRILOGY

"Nicholas Pearson is one of the most plainly knowledgeable mineral persons I have met in my life. He masterfully bridges the worlds of the head and the heart, along with corresponding rituals. The crystal adventure is just beginning. Read this book and you will walk in both those worlds, and your life will be forever enriched—likely enchanted."

MARILYN TWINTREESS, COAUTHOR OF THE
STONES ALIVE! TRILOGY, FEEDING THE LIVING BODY AND SOUL,
AND ELEMENTAL BIRTH IMPRINTS

"A deep and thorough exploration of seven power stone spirits. Rather than just list the properties of the stones, Nicholas Pearson uses the history, myth, and science of the stones to create experiences that allow you to directly engage with their energies and spiritual lessons. I thoroughly enjoyed this book and learned some new things about some old favorite stones."

CHRISTOPHER PENCZAK, AUTHOR OF THE
TEMPLE OF WITCHCRAFT SERIES

THE SEVEN
ARCHETYPAL
STONES

THEIR SPIRITUAL
POWERS AND TEACHINGS

NICHOLAS PEARSON

Destiny Books
Rochester, Vermont • Toronto, Canada

Destiny Books
One Park Street
Rochester, Vermont 05767
www.DestinyBooks.com

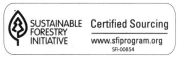

Text stock is SFI certified

Destiny Books is a division of Inner Traditions International

Library of Congress Cataloging-in-Publication Data
Names: Pearson, Nicholas, 1986– author.
Title: The seven archetypal stones : their spiritual powers and teachings / Nicholas Pearson.
Description: Rochester, Vermont : Destiny Books, [2016] | Includes bibliographical references and index.
Identifiers: LCCN 2016016623 (print) | LCCN 2016023314 (e-book) | ISBN 9781620555477 (paperback) | ISBN 9781620555484 (e-book)
Subjects: LCSH: Crystals--Therapeutic use. | Stone--Therapeutic use. | Mind and body. | BISAC: BODY, MIND & SPIRIT / Crystals. | BODY, MIND & SPIRIT / Healing / Energy (Chi Kung, Reiki, Polarity). | HEALTH & FITNESS / Alternative Therapies.
Classification: LCC RZ415 .P43 2016 (print) | LCC RZ415 (e-book) | DDC 615.8/52--dc23
LC record available at https://lccn.loc.gov/2016016623

Printed and bound in the United States by Lake Book Manufacturing, Inc. The text stock is SFI certified. The Sustainable Forestry Initiative® program promotes sustainable forest management.

10   9   8   7   6   5   4   3   2   1

Text design and layout by Virginia Scott Bowman
This book was typeset in Garamond with Trajan Sans used as the display typeface

To send correspondence to the author of this book, mail a first-class letter to the author c/o Inner Traditions • Bear & Company, One Park Street, Rochester, VT 05767, and we will forward the communication.

This book is dedicated to my late grandfather, Ron Pearson. His gift of my very first piece of quartz transformed me from the young boy who picked up rocks as souvenirs into a lover of fine minerals; this was the first time I experienced the alchemy offered by the crystalline kingdom. This piece of rock crystal sits beside me, even today. His greatest gift, however, was unconditional love and support in my childhood and adolescent years, which helped me find my voice and gave me the courage to share my passion with the world. Thank you for planting the seeds that would shape my life.

CONTENTS

ACKNOWLEDGMENTS

It would be an insurmountable task to personally acknowledge everyone who helped this project become a reality, so I shall attempt to name the key players and beg forgiveness to anyone not listed below. All of my friends and loved ones have been amazingly supportive and helpful for the duration of this process.

To my partner, Steven Walsh, I owe you gratitude for your support in ways I never imagined could be given. Thank you for your photographic and artistic expertise in this and subsequent texts. Thank you for supporting major life changes that led me to writing and publishing. And, of course, thank you for loving me in spite of the bouts of lunacy and messiness that were born of my creative process. My sincerest love and humblest gratitude may never be enough to repay you.

To my best friend, Kathy Moyer, I cannot say thank you enough; you have been my biggest cheerleader and the first person to review my early work. My gratitude for all your love, support, and honest feedback could never be measured.

To my family near and far, I offer my gratitude for more than I can include here. Without your love and acceptance, this chapter of my life would be less fulfilling. It is a blessing to have your support in my endeavors, no matter how different the path might be from the original plan. I love you all dearly, and this book couldn't have been written without the ups and downs of growing together.

To Brandon Weltz, your gift of believing in me when no one else did left an indelible mark on my soul. Thank you for the many years of adventure and for helping me make connections that have brought me into my own. I will be forever appreciative that the Master Gardener placed us in the same garden plot with our extended, co-created family. To the rest of this family, thank you for teaching me the values of community, responsibility, and compassion. I am indebted to your kindness and help through the past decade of my life.

To Rita Truax and Patricia Williams, special acknowledgments are due. In my late teen years you saw in me a potential I didn't see in myself. Thank you for inviting me to teach in your stores and for teaching me so many lessons over the years. To the rest of my amazing hosts and all of my students over the past twelve years, working with you is literally a dream come true. Without an opportunity to share my love of the mineral kingdom with you, I could never have made it this far in life.

To the past and present staff of the Gillespie Museum at Stetson University, thank you for enabling me to expand my love for rocks and minerals through a deeper appreciation of earth science. For allowing me to thrive among the treasures of the earth I will always be deeply grateful.

Finally, I send my gratitude to the staff of Inner Traditions. Everyone I've connected with has been delightful and helpful. Thank you Erica Robinson for chatting with me and inviting me to send in my incomplete text; I don't know that I would have followed through with finishing the book without your encouragement. Thank you to Jon Graham for believing in the potential of this work and offering me a place among the talented family of authors published through Inner Traditions. And to my editor, Jamaica Burns, thank you for your expertise, patience, and willingness to help a first-time author.

Introduction

The mineral kingdom, comprised of beautiful crystals, dense rocks, sand, clay, and everything in between, is the very foundation of life on Earth. The rocks and minerals of our beloved planet form the very ground on which we walk and surround us in daily life. Metals are refined from ores and provide the structural framework for buildings, cars, and innumerable quotidian objects; glass is smelted from silica and ash and provides us with another structural material and countless other things we take for granted; gypsum is ever-present in modern life, on everything from plaster, to blackboard chalk, to wallboard. We are literally inseparable from the crystallinity of the planet.

THE ROLE OF CRYSTALS
IN OUR LIVES

Humankind has been fascinated with rocks since the discovery of tools and the subsequent creation of ornaments. Cutting edges and projectiles, as well as pounding tools and weights, may have been the first known use of rocks. However, at some point one of our early ancestors must have picked up a stone just because its appearance was beguiling, or maybe even for a more nebulous quality: the way it *felt*. The history of minerals as ornaments and ritual implements is as old as human history. The relationship between humans and minerals is chronicled in artifacts from every culture that has ever walked the earth.

Today, not only do science, technology, and industry utilize the rich storehouse of mineral wealth, healers and mystics collect and revere the spiritual worth of gemstones and crystals. Encyclopedias and other books extolling their properties fill bookshelves; workshops attract attendees eager to explore the nature of crystals. The ancient call to co-create with the mineral kingdom lives on in an unbroken legacy, even into the twenty-first century.

Each year, new mineral deposits are found, some containing familiar stones while others surprise us with previously unknown beauties. Psychics and sensitives provide insight into their energies, and they are then cataloged alongside thousands of extant varieties of healing stones. The very same impetus to explore, categorize, and utilize the power of crystals has existed for centuries. With each passing year there are new developments in the understanding and use of crystals and minerals, and thus crystal healers become better equipped to alleviate the ills of the world. Simultaneously, as advances in the science of mineralogy occur, our understanding of the mineral kingdom becomes more profound.

The aim of my life's work has always been to unite these two seemingly disparate and opposing forces. Spirit and science can work together to improve our relationship with minerals, with each field informing the other. Over the years, as my personal work and teachings have evolved, I've begun to call this approach "ethnogeology." It is an interdisciplinary approach, one that looks at how humankind and the mineral kingdom interact on all levels: scientific, biological, environmental, ornamental, spiritual. It's not a hard science; instead, it requires sensitivity and intuition, just like any other healing art.

This book is meant to help you expand your work with crystals. Rather than merely providing yet another encyclopedia that discusses the properties specific to different mineral formations, this work is intended to help the reader look deeper than just the surface level. Crystals work at archetypal levels, and understanding their mission and characteristic energies can open our eyes to stones in new and exciting ways.

WHY ARCHETYPES?

An archetype is a prototype of sorts. It is the measuring stick for everything that is modeled in its form. Archetypes serve as the original blueprints, the master molds, the perfected state for any concept. Crystal archetypes are the ideals that the stones themselves represent, either through human application or through an exploration of their structure and composition. Crystal archetypes are teachers, and their lessons are based on a lineage that is as old as time itself.

When exploring the crystal archetypes, there are two main varieties. The *explicate archetypes* are those modeled after historical, evidence-based examples of the use of a particular stone from culture to culture. In some sense they should be universal, that is, the symbolic messages should not be so narrow as to be completely alien to any culture outside of which they are found. They can be simple artifacts, such as obsidian arrowheads, or mythological representations etched in stone, such as jade dragons.

The second variety of crystal archetypes is the *implicate archetype.* The message of these archetypes must be decoded through the layers of symbolism inherent in artifacts, morphology, composition, and myth. Implicate archetypes may not have a physical counterpart among the relics of ancient people. Instead, an appreciation for mineral science often lends a clearer understanding of these archetypes. They are the ideals encoded within the stones themselves.

Looking at the different stones through such an intensely focused lens can provide a level of intimacy with each mineral not found in other books written about all things crystalline. The goal here is to look at the world of rocks and minerals as a kind of mystery school where those who choose to listen closely to the original mystery tradition of this planet are initiated. Each gemstone explored in this text serves to help unfold one's spiritual path by accessing certain universal truths.

Because the nature of exploring the archetypes is so in-depth, the scope of this work is limited to just seven stones. They have been selected based on such factors as their availability, the ubiquity of their usage, and the depth of spiritual meaning latent in each gemstone. Truly, it would be a monumental undertaking to give similar treatments to even a dozen stones, so these seven were selected for the clarity of their messages and the impact they make on the lives of anyone who chooses to work with them.

The archetypes teach through form, symbol, and story. Although each entry can be viewed as a complete teaching, most of the messages of the minerals themselves build on one another. When strung together they become a series of instructions that serve to initiate the seeker into the mystery tradition of the mineral kingdom itself. Thus learning from the stones offers a means of spiritual development. Truly, there is no destination, no endpoint; there is only the path. Connecting with the crystal archetypes may reveal the direction of the path, but it is up to the reader to take the first step by becoming immersed in this knowledge.

HOW TO USE THIS BOOK

This book has been written with every level of proficiency and a multitude of applications in mind. For those interested in history, archaeology, and mythology, the tales told by the artifacts will both entertain and educate. Crystal therapists and healers of any level of expertise will be able to find new methods for harnessing the power of the mineral kingdom for personal or professional practices. Spiritual seekers and aspirants can find guideposts along the path through the descriptions of the archetypes themselves.

Each chapter in this book opens with a geological and historical perspective of the specific gemstone under review. This serves as the foundation for understanding the how and why of each archetype. After gaining this basic understanding, the archetype of the stone is introduced. Each archetype has at least one accompanying exercise or meditation. These activities are designed to be simple, practical, and effective. They can be practiced as often as you like, with or without regard to the order in which they are presented. Generally, the earlier exercises are building blocks for those occurring later, although each is a stand-alone undertaking.

Prior to each exercise or meditation it is suggested that you cleanse whichever stone you are working with. This can be done through a variety of methods. Sacred sound can be used, such as chanting, singing bowls, toning, or other sounds to which you are drawn. The smoke of sage or other herbs and incenses can also be employed for cleansing your beloved crystalline tools, and many practitioners prefer sunlight, moonlight, sea salt, or water for cleansing. The options are seemingly endless. Since many rocks and minerals can be bleached in sunlight, scratched by salt, or otherwise damaged by water, I prefer to use consciousness-based methods, such as the following.

EXERCISE

CLEANSING YOUR STONE

Before cleansing your stone, spend a moment or two setting your intention and quieting the mind. Grasp your stone between the thumb and index finger of your dominant hand; if this is uncomfortable, larger specimens may instead be cradled in the palm of one or both hands. Take several deep, rhythmic breaths while establishing a connection to the stone. Imagine that you are breathing in white light. Take a deep breath, filling your entire being with this white light; exhale with a single, powerful pulse of air through the nose. Picture your exhalation carrying the white light to your chosen stone, sweeping away any disharmonious energy, leaving behind a clean slate.

Finally, I include detailed information on how the stone can be applied in crystal healing practice. Sources from ancient to modern are included, and their relevance to the archetypal messages of the minerals is emphasized so that the reader can gain a clear perspective on the how and why of it all. This section on healing is particularly useful for anyone seeking to find a practical application for crystals in the context of a therapeutic practice.

Following the discourse on healing properties, a short compendium of subvarieties and related stones is included. In most cases this list includes minerals that are compositionally or morphologically similar. In the case of some of the more precious gemstones such as diamond and emerald, the list includes affordable substitutes that connect to those stones' archetypes. These lists allow the reader to explore more than just the seven stones included in this book, while still adhering to the themes presented in each chapter.

It is my sincere hope that this book will help you, the reader, with your personal growth and healing. Since before recorded history the messages of the mineral kingdom have nurtured and initiated many changes on both the global and the personal scale. As the earth and its inhabitants continue to evolve, especially on the spiritual level, new tools are necessary to sustain this process. Thankfully, new tools *are* available to us, in the form of the earth's oldest mentors: the members of the mineral kingdom.

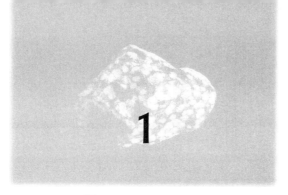

OBSIDIAN

The Spear and the Mirror

Dark as the void of space and reflective as a polished mirror, obsidian has long fascinated humankind. This midnight black stone is volcanic in origin, a natural glass that originates when silica-rich lava cools too quickly for crystallization to occur. Obsidian's name is credited to its discoverer, the Roman explorer Obsius, who is thought to have first encountered this mineraloid in Ethiopia.[1] For some prehistoric cultures it was the prime material for knapping into blades and points for projectiles; for others it served as a magic mirror into other realms. In healing practice today it can serve as a stone of initiation, for its fiery birth can help us become reborn, and its sharp edges can cut away the obstacles in our path while granting insight and clear vision.

Obsidian is an amorphous solid; really, it is just a super-cooled liquid that as a glass lacks the long-range order that characterizes true minerals. Its composition is mostly silica, but the rapid nature of its cooling process prevents its constituent compounds from ordering themselves into neatly organized, regular structures. Obsidian is therefore disqualified from being counted as a true mineral because of its lack of crystalline structure. Although under close magnification obsidian shows evidence of short-range order—minute clusters of molecules that began to arrange themselves in crystal-like ways—these groupings do not add up to a complete crystal lattice. This incompleteness is part of obsidian's beauty; it has one foot in the realm of the mineral kingdom and the other in the void of becoming.

Obsidian is found in regions with volcanic activity, as felsic lava is the parent material to this rock. Some notable occurrences include Central and South America (including Mexico, Argentina, and Peru), as well as the Southwest and Northwest United States, New Zealand, Japan, Iceland, Kenya, Canada, and Armenia. While most obsidian varieties appear to be black, there are several other varieties found worldwide, including snowflake obsidian, mahogany obsidian, and rainbow obsidian, as well as a type that produces a metallic sheen when polished. Most varieties show a translucent or transparent greenish color when sliced thin and held to the light. Rarely, deposits of gem-quality obsidian can be found, with green to brown gemstones being the most common; bluish green, yellowish, and gray colors have been confirmed too.

The chemical makeup and nature of obsidian's structure endow it with a brittle hardness and conchoidal fracture. Ancient cultures made use of these properties to craft sharp edges that were ideal for cutting tools and arrowheads. Obsidian was a favored tool for cutting because of the sharpness and sureness of the blade. By knapping obsidian in the same manner as flint was worked, fine tools were created for both secular and sacred uses. Obsidian arrowheads, spearpoints, knives, and scrapers can be found in many parts of the world, including Turkey, Egypt, throughout the Americas, and New Zealand.

As lapidary skills developed beyond flint knapping, ornaments made of obsidian became available. Beads, effigies, and other adornments could be crafted from this material with greater ease. Eventually, this led to the ability to finely polish obsidian, and its smooth, dark surface was prized for use as a mirror because it showed only the shadowy forms underlying what was reflected in it. Some cultures polished rounded spheres in addition to mirrors, while the native people of New Zealand used inlaid obsidian in the eyes of their statues.

Cultures that encountered obsidian often wove myths around its unusual occurrence and appearance and held it in high esteem for spiritual uses. In ancient Mexico, obsidian was known as *ixtli,* after the deity Tezcatlipoca, whose name means "smoking mirror" or "shining mirror." Mirrors carved from obsidian are one of the most iconic Mesoamerican uses of this igneous rock. Because an obsidian mirror reflects merely the shadows of the objects and people held before it, it was believed to connect to the afterlife, and its supernatural correspondence created a link to divination. Obsidian became associated with death, the underworld, and second sight. Accordingly, vases and mirrors of obsidian have been found among other funerary offerings in Mexico.[2] Masks carved from obsidian and used for funerary purposes have similarly been discovered throughout Teotihuacan.[3]

A variety of obsidian known as "Pele's hair," after the Polynesian goddess of creation, who is often associated with volcanoes, is found as fibers or threads of volcanic glass often golden brown in color. This variety is typically found downwind of volcanic vents. Pele rules over the underworld, and as in many shamanic and mythological traditions, this is where the souls of the dead are believed to dwell. Some modern mystics believe that Pele releases the souls of the dead with her volcanic eruptions, permitting them to be reborn and continue the cycle of reincarnation; although Native Hamaiians do not traditionally subscribe to reincarnation.[4]

Apache tears, a variety of obsidian that surrounds the translucent to transparent nodules found in a perlite matrix, also has mythic origins. This variety is found in the American Southwest, where it is said to have formed when warriors of this Native American tribe were defeated in battle. The grief of the mourning women was said to have been so great that their tears hardened into stone when they fell to the ground, thus birthing the obsidian nodules. The legend maintains that anyone in possession of an Apache tear will never cry again.[5]

OBSIDIAN AS AN ARCHETYPE:
THE SPEAR

The earliest known use of obsidian in human civilization is in the form of blades and projectiles. Arrowheads and spearpoints are easily knapped from obsidian due to its brittle structure, and the conchoidal fracture yields a deft cutting edge. The word *conchoidal* is derived from the Greek root word for *mussel,* referring to the curved, broken surface left when mechanical stress is applied to materials such as flint, obsidian, and quartz. By controlling the impact, stones can be worked into tools with sharp cutting edges. In areas where obsidian is present, native people used it as a tool in both mundane and sacred activities. Evidence shows that obsidian tools were used especially among Mesoamerican cultures in ritual sacrifice and bloodletting, while many warriors and hunters around the world used obsidian projectiles to hunt and to prepare food and to fight battles.

The archetype of obsidian as the spear or blade represents the archetype of the warrior. The warrior teaches us that we must undergo a transformation wherein we claim our power. The first stage of this metamorphosis is an internal one, as we begin to change our attitudes about the blows we are dealt in life. Just as a raw piece of obsidian is gradually transformed into a blade as the flint knapper strikes again and again, so are we also molded and sculpted by life. Trauma, pain, and suffering can be tools to refine our consciousness if we give ourselves the opportunity to apply them as such. Each time we feel as though life has knocked us down, it is an opportunity to use that state to surrender to the process of becoming.

Flake by flake, the raw stone is chipped away and the point is revealed. In our own lives, obsidian helps us to be more present through pain and to surrender to the process unfolding. When we hold obsidian or meditate with it during times of transition, we can access the stillness in our being that is capable of weathering any storm. When we offer resistance, we are clinging to the shards of our lives that appear to be broken off rather than seeing the transformation that is occurring. Obsidian asks us not to look at the broken pieces lying on the ground; rather, this stone helps us to see ourselves as the perfection that is revealed from within when the unnecessary parts of ourselves are stripped away. Only by surrendering to the mystery of the process, by allowing Source to slowly help us release that which no longer serves us, can we become complete. Every piece we lose in this process is really just part of our false identity, the ego, which is gradually broken down and left behind. Through the stages of breaking down and chipping away, our authentic self, hidden beneath the surface, is revealed.

Obsidian has long been touted for having a protective and shielding influence. It is often carried to defend against psychic attack as well as to shield the holder from disruptive environmental influences, whether they are present spiritually, mentally, or physically. As we embrace the energy of the warrior, we find less of a need to create barriers between ourselves and the rest of the world. The role of the spiritual warrior is to accept responsibility and accountability for one's actions and to defend the light of the world. Obsidian serves to arm the spiritual warrior with a tool that cuts through illusion and pain. The sharpness that is typical of obsidian endows us with a mental attitude that is similarly penetrative, and this helps cut through the allure of the material world and those who are ruled by it.

Ancient arrowheads of any material have been known by many names, from "thunder stones" to "elf shot," and they have long been esteemed as protective amulets. Wearing or carrying such artifacts was believed to deflect negative energies and protect against the fairy folk. The fairy folk are beings that dwell in a plane that is more or less parallel to our own; it exists within and beyond the world we know. Fairies are known by many names across the world and are traditionally associated with the forces of nature. Some of these beings are considered mischievous and others are even malevolent, so ancient peoples often sought protection from those that may have caused trouble.

Metaphorically, obsidian projectiles help us to take aim in life and to shoot down any obstacles in our path. When we embrace our true power, embodying the archetype of the warrior, we are able to surmount anything standing in our way. In crystal healing, blades and spearpoints can be used to cut through energetic cords or attachments; in meditation they may be employed as a symbolic means of casting off attachments to ego and mind.

The spear is definitely a rugged archetype. One might ask why this is the first aspect to be explored, as on the surface this quality does not seem to correlate to any particular mystery-school teachings. The archetype of the spear is at first very externally focused. It helps to find direction and cut off distracting influences. Because of this outward focus, the true state of being is more easily achieved. As we recognize each time that life strikes at our raw form as a step along the path of becoming our true self, we can take that external awareness and shift it within the self. By our embracing the only real power as coming from the divine, surrender becomes the most powerful state of being possible.

The spear gives us the courage and the power to strip away those parts of ourselves that weigh us down. When we can honestly look at our life and recognize a behavior or choice that does not serve our highest purpose, we can cut it out and hand it over to the Higher Power. This is the ultimate message of the blade used in sacrificial rites: by offering our hearts willingly and authentically, we are given the opportunity to release what isn't working and receive true strength. No illusion originating in the material world can survive this strength.

MEDITATION

HONING YOUR STRENGTH

Obsidian has been used for eons as a tool to ensure safety and strength, as its energy conveys protection and grounding. The path of the spiritual warrior is to harness obsidian's strength through surrender. This meditation eases one's mind and heart, allowing us to embrace the moments when life feels as though it is knocking us down. It can be practiced proactively to build strength, but it is an especially great remedy for the experience of pain or anxiety as growth opportunities arise.

To begin, select a piece of obsidian; I prefer an arrowhead or raw, broken obsidian with a sharp edge. Before beginning the following meditation, cleanse your obsidian. Stand with your feet shoulder-width apart in a powerful warrior stance. Take a couple of deep breaths to begin to relax. Note where tension dwells in your body. Hold your obsidian to your solar plexus, the third chakra that lies just below the breastbone, with both hands keeping it in place. This chakra is the seat of power, and obsidian fortifies it.

As you stand with the obsidian in place, breathe rhythmically into the belly in such a manner that the solar plexus gently expands and contracts with each breath in and out. Allow your mind to call the source of fear, pain, or worry. As you begin to feel the tug of these emotions, breathe into the obsidian and surrender to the moment. Know that this moment, with all its challenges, is an opportunity to sharpen your mind and your focus. Lean into the discomfort and uncertainty and remain grounded through the stone. As you recognize the authentic source of discomfort as uncertainty, the familiar tension in your body will begin to dissipate. Accept the strength that comes from being fully present in the state of surrender. Ask Source for guidance if you still feel uncertain, and know that it will be provided.

When you feel centered and at ease, bring the obsidian to your heart chakra, at the center of the chest, and offer gratitude to the stone and to the universe. To overcome a specific obstacle, this meditation may also be partnered with the cord-cutting ritual described later in this chapter (see pages 29–30).

OBSIDIAN AS AN ARCHETYPE: THE MIRROR

This volcanic glass is best known among students of the magical and cultural arts for its use as a medium for divination: the mirror. Obsidian easily takes a high polish, and when made smooth, this dark stone is highly reflective. The images seen on its surface are dark and shadowy, and they point to the notion that spiritual truth cannot be found in the forms of anything in the material world.

The importance accorded mirrors in ancient cultures offers a glimpse at certain universal spiritual ideals. In his seminal work *The Four Agreements,* Don Miguel Ruiz describes a Toltec concept called *mitote,* which is the mental chatter and noise that keeps us from seeing the nature of creation as being a reflection of the light of Creator. Everything that exists is really light at its core, and what we see here in the physical world is really just a reflection of that light. We must learn to see it in ourselves and in others, as well as in all parts of creation. In so doing, we clear the space between the mirrors in order to see that light reflected. If the level of true existence is a plane of light, then the dream that we experience here in the physical world is, according to Toltec wisdom, a world of smoke that clouds the light and prevents us from seeing who we really are.

Mitote, therefore, could be considered to be the smoke between the mirrors. If each human being heart can reflect the nature of reality as the light of the spiritual plane, then the mental chatter of mitote forms as smoke between these heart-mirrors, occluding the images being reflected from one to the next. It is the role of the spiritual aspirant to more clearly reflect spiritual truth in all of his or her thoughts and deeds. To do this requires a great deal of inner work, work that frees the self of the ego-held belief that we belong to the world of the smoke between the mirrors. We must learn to see through this smoke in order to see our true self, which is one with Creator and is reflected in all of life and all of existence. The flipside of this is that we must also spend time polishing the mirror of our heart in order to better reflect this truth to those who gaze into it.

The mirror is used by many cultures to represent a divine connection. In Shinto, the native religion of Japan, the sun goddess Amaterasu is represented by ornate mirrors, and one such mirror is a component of Japan's legendary Imperial Regalia (also known as the Three Sacred Treasures of Japan). Mirrors were symbols of truth in premodern Japan, and they factor into a number of myths and influenced the arts there. My favorite evidence of the mirror as a spiritual metaphor is from a poem by Emperor Meiji (1852–1912), very simply titled "Kagami," or "mirror": "I (even if I am the emperor) will polish the mirror of my mind further, learning from ordinary people who have a wonderful clarity of mind."[6] The act of polishing the mirror of one's mind returns again and again as we look further into obsidian's symbolism. It is noteworthy that the Japanese language uses the same word to signify both the heart and the mind, which brings us to the recognition that the effects of obsidian as a mirror bridge the two. Seeking the truth of who we really are as reflected to us in the hearts of others bridges the cultural divide, as exemplified in this bit of Japanese poetry.

Mirrors are also a branch of the family tree of the "theology of light," which is to say that there is a widespread use of light imagery and optical symbolism central to nearly all of the world's religions and spiritual beliefs, which we will explore further in subsequent chapters. What is of great interest to us with regard to obsidian is not the optical quality of the stone, because it doesn't actually reflect light well enough to produce a clear, vibrant image. Instead, it only shows the *shadows* of the forms, thereby granting access to the realms that are hidden below the world of form.

Obsidian mirrors have been made famous through their discovery at pre-Columbian archeological sites. These sacred objects were made in honor of the god Tezcatlipoca and his analogs in other Mesoamerican cultures. Tezcatlipoca rules over the night sky, hurricanes, war, divination, jaguars, and the earth. He is sometimes depicted in effigies carved from obsidian, or as obsidian mirrors themselves. This deity was one of the four central creator gods in Aztec mythology, and his priests employed polished specimens of obsidian to achieve trance states, to offer healing, and to receive intuitive guidance. Additionally, priests of the god of the smoking mirror made use of sharpened obsidian blades for bloodletting and sacrifices.

These mirrors later became popular among occultists and magicians in Europe. Scrying, the art of divination by gazing into a more or less reflective surface, became popular among the learned class during the sixteenth century as obsidian mirrors from Mexico made their way into the hands of some notable practitioners, including the advisor to Queen Elizabeth I, Dr. John Dee. A tool such as this was often referred to as a "shew-stone," or speculum. Magic mirrors have maintained their popularity among some schools of Western occultists to this day.

The obsidian mirror serves to tap into the subconscious mind as we allow our relaxed gaze to fix on its surface. Scrying works by allowing the eyes to defocus and the mind to unwind; images may be seen on the surface of the speculum or in the mind's eye. Obsidian is a tool par excellence for this activity because its dark, gleaming surface helps us penetrate the veil between the worlds. This volcanic glass has gathered a number of supernatural associations, and it is born from a natural phenomenon that was once little understood. This places it within the context of other such phenomena, which were often relegated to the realms of myth, magic, and the supernatural.

EXERCISE

LEARNING TO SCRY

Divination is the process of seeking intuitive guidance, and it can make use of any number of tools. Cultures around the world have used natural bodies of water, vessels filled with water, a variety of gemstones and rocks, smoke, fire, ink, and numerous other mediums to scry. For this exercise, we will use a polished specimen of obsidian such as an obsidian mirror. The obsidian serves as a connection into the subconscious, the void of becoming. By connecting us to the universe this way, obsidian catalyzes the process of receiving intuitive messages. Simultaneously, the relaxed gaze employed in this technique helps shut down the chatter of the conscious mind, thereby making it easier for the subconscious, or soul consciousness, to be heard and seen readily.

To have an effective scrying session, ensure that you will remain undisturbed. Cleanse and consecrate your obsidian mirror prior to use. A dimly lit atmosphere best lends itself to scrying, and many diviners prefer to use candlelight to illumine their space. Avoid having reflections of the source of light fall directly on the surface of the obsidian. Before commencing, I usually like to create sacred space and invite the presence of the divine and any guides, angels, or ascended beings who are willing participate in creating the highest good.

Scrying can address specific questions, or it may be left open-ended in order to bring insight to whichever situation is at hand. Historically, this form of divination was used for shedding light not only on the future but also on the past and present. Select your focus, and ask obsidian to guide you to the messages you wish to receive. It's generally good to keep some paper and a pen or pencil nearby to jot down notes for later interpretation.

To begin, stare into the surface of your obsidian mirror. Rather than merely looking at the reflections produced, stare beyond the surface by gently unfocusing your eyes. Let your mind become still and pay attention to any images, symbols, or thoughts that are raised by the subconscious. You may view these as images on or in the mirror, or you may perceive them in your mind's eye. Both experiences are valid. Be mindful of the images and take notes as you proceed or immediately upon finishing the session. Remember, the subconscious communicates in symbols that will likely require interpretation, which is why it is good to take notes. To end, simply extend your gratitude to the stone and refocus your eyes.

Scrying requires practice to achieve results. Do not be disappointed if you receive no images on your initial attempts. Continue to practice until you receive results. Divination, as a general rule, does not give us absolute predictions; the guidance received through this or any other divinatory vehicle is merely offering a most likely outcome or path. Any number of decisions we make can alter this path, so you can use this information to make informed decisions and attain success in life.

Reflecting the True Self

In crystal healing, obsidian is a stone for shadow work. It can reveal the root cause underlying physical, mental, or emotional illness and distress. A powerful healer, this volcanic rock is described by crystal healer and author Katrina Raphaell as "one of the most important teachers of all the New Age Stones."[7] She goes on to describe the effects of black obsidian, saying that it "acts as a mirror that reflects the flaws in one's nature and magnifies the fears, insecurities, and egocentric attitudes that suppress the soul's superior qualities."[8] Through working with any form of obsidian, light is shined into the dark places, and we are able to resolve our fears by facing them head-on.

The archetype of the mirror is one that appeals to the nature of what is reflected. Since obsidian shows a shadowy image reflected on its surface, it taps into the shadows of our mind. Obsidian's dark color takes us beneath the surface of our being and permits us to confront whatever we find. The dark color and lack of crystal structure provides a link to the state of uncertainty; many times what is reflected to us by obsidian is our potential for vulnerability. This sentiment serves as the tipping point for many of us who hide our vulnerability in order to avoid fear, shame, and uncertainty. However, this vulnerable state, when embraced, is also the source of positive, uplifting emotions. Vulnerability researcher Brené Brown writes that vulnerability is "the birthplace of love, belonging, joy, courage, empathy, and creativity. It is the source of hope, empathy, accountability, and authenticity. If we want greater clarity in our purpose or deeper and more meaningful spiritual lives, vulnerability is the path."[9] When given the right perspective by obsidian, we are able to fully and honestly see and reconcile our emotions.

Iztli, as obsidian was known to the Aztecs, was fashioned into images of Tezcatlipoca, whose very name points to one of the benefits of working with obsidian. As we face our fears and embrace our power through surrender, the smoke between the mirrors begins to clear. This allows our light to shine more brightly and increases our range of vision. This will, in turn, inspire others to see the light reflected in the mirrors of their hearts. In the works of the forerunners of today's crystal-healing movement, obsidian is often regarded as a stone that is not for the faint of heart. It is regarded as a gemstone whose energies are intense and honest. We see that "consulting the mirror is the option to see the repressed part of ourselves and to give feeling to that which is difficult to integrate."[10] Obsidian's nature as a catalyst for releasing our fears can lead us to the understanding of the biggest fear of all. Marianne Williamson best describes this fear in her best-selling book *A Return to Love:*

> Our deepest fear is not that we are inadequate. Our deepest fear is that we are powerful beyond measure. It is our light, not our darkness that most frightens us. We ask ourselves, Who am I to be brilliant, gorgeous, talented, fabulous? Actually, who are you not to be? You are a child of God. Your playing small does not serve the world. There is nothing enlightened about shrinking so that other people won't feel insecure around you. We are all meant to shine, as children do. We were born to make manifest the glory of God that is within us. It's not just in some of us; it's in everyone. And as we let our own light shine, we unconsciously give other people permission to do the same. As we are liberated from our own fear, our presence automatically liberates others.[11]

A polished piece of obsidian symbolizes the next stage after the spearpoint. If the cutting edges require the percussive action of the flint knapper, the mirror requires the patience and precision of a lapidary artist. The rough shape must be transformed from a primal tool into an elegant objet d'art. The action is akin to the notion of polishing the mirror of our hearts; only through repeated motions against the turning wheel will the rough stone be given a reflective surface. We can learn to harness this patience as we do our inner work.

What I have found in my own healing work and in observing the work of others is that too often we recognize that there is a part of ourselves that we need to look at with integrity and candor in order to release it, but we are afraid to do so. This fear generally announces itself as shame, and we will sidestep our vulnerability in order to avoid the disempowering nature of shame. The mirror, incorrectly used, might appear to be a reflective shield, and it can be used to hide our fears from us as well as to deflect unwanted probing from external influences. The problem with this is that without the strength of the warrior, we cannot withstand too many blows from behind the obsidian shield.

By its very nature obsidian is brittle and will break. The jagged edges will only result in more pain, so it is imperative not to misuse the archetype of the mirror. Holding the mirror up is not a means of chasing away the things that frighten us or a way of fending off our own destructive thought patterns; our mirrors are not meant to shield us from the light and darkness around us. Rather, they are powerful tools that reflect what is within. Acceptance of one's vulnerability and a willingness to understand shame are necessary stepping stones to wholeness. For this reason, we have accepted the archetype of the spear first. Imagine going into a dark place unprepared or unarmed. Uncertainty is one of the most profoundly unsettling emotions, but having the tools to cope with it, such as your ego-cutting spearpoint and mirror for seeing into the unknown, will help you cross the boundaries into uncertainty in order to release fear, shame, resentment, and doubt.

Obsidian encourages us to not just look within but to integrate what we find and heal it. This is the premise behind bringing the darkness into the light. All our fears, worries, and resentments are a result of our attachments, and we learn from many spiritual traditions that attachment is the root of suffering. We can cut the cords of attachment and polish what lies beneath them. In this way, we begin to refine our inner mirror such that we can better reflect our innate state of perfection. As we do so, our shining light inspires others. This is the true meaning of Emperor Meiji's poem: we do not work to better ourselves for the sake of fame or fortune; instead, as we focus on becoming whole for the sake of doing our part to help the world, others are spurred toward self-actualization. In this way the smoke between the mirrors clears bit by bit.

MEDITATION

SEEING THE SHADOW

Obsidian's mirrorlike qualities can be harnessed to reveal the hidden aspects of oneself that need to be brought into the light in order to become whole. In this exercise, obsidian grants access to the hidden parts of your being, and its energy can be directed toward embracing the shadow side for integration and healing.

To do this meditation you may either sit and gaze into a polished piece of obsidian, or you can meditate lying down with a piece of obsidian resting at the third eye, between and slightly above the eyebrows. I find rainbow obsidian and snowflake obsidian to be especially helpful during this exercise, although any dark variety will suffice. As before, cleanse your obsidian before proceeding. Breathe deeply and begin to relax. As your mind connects with the frequency of obsidian, ask for guidance and protection from the divine, using whichever language is comfortable for you. Visualize yourself surrounded by a protective sphere of obsidian, then turn your gaze inward.

Silently state your intention; ask that obsidian guide you to one of your shadow aspects. This may show up as a painful or traumatic memory, or perhaps as some secret you try to keep your conscious mind and ego from seeing. When an image or memory materializes in your mind's eye, accept what you see without judgment. Obsidian may show the broken pieces of oneself that are buried far beneath the surface, and it can be unrelenting.

Breathe into the experience and send love and forgiveness to your shadow self. Begin a dialogue with what you see before you and ask for additional help from the Higher Power if any part of the process brings discomfort. At this point, speak to the self you see before you and tell this part of your shadow that you love it, for you could not be where you are today without it. Call on the strength of your inner warrior to be vulnerable to your shadow self and to integrate it lovingly.

After offering healing words to reconcile your shadow, move the obsidian to your heart chakra, located in the center of the chest, and envision your shadow self moving into the light of your heart. Thank your shadow for being part of your journey and for providing an opportunity for healing. As it enters the light, feel that its darkness is transmuted into light. Breathe deeply with your obsidian cradled at your heart until you feel wholeness growing within.

You can repeat this process to heal other pieces of your shadow self, or you may conclude your meditation. To do so, thank the Higher Power that you invoked, as well as thanking your shadow and obsidian too. Allow the obsidian shield around you to dissipate, and send its energy into the earth to be recycled. When finished, open your eyes and cleanse the obsidian used for this meditation.

OBSIDIAN AS AN ARCHETYPE: THE VOID

Early in the discussion of obsidian's composition and formation it was established that this volcanic rock is noncrystalline. Years ago I spent time working in an earth-science museum that was home to one of the largest historical mineral collections in the Southeast. Those days in the museum nurtured in me an even deeper love for the mineral kingdom, and it gave the impetus for me to combine spiritual insights with scientific facts. One of my greatest fascinations has been with the seven crystal systems, which are the classifications of the symmetries expressed by minerals. I spent countless hours looking for the parallels between the energy of crystals and their internal and external geometries.

As noted earlier, obsidian does not fit into any of the seven crystal systems because it lacks a crystalline structure. As an amorphous solid it cannot be bound by axes of symmetry or form crystal faces. The conditions under which it is formed are rapid and spontaneous: lava quickly erupts and cools before it can permit its constituents to precipitate as crystalline structures in host rock. Because obsidian is created very rapidly, especially when compared to most rocks and minerals, its birth often resembles chaos incarnate.

In many traditions worldwide it is said that the universe was created from a primordial void. This void was pregnant with possibilities, but it lacked the order and structure of creation. Today, science echoes this idea with its theory about the state of the universe before the Big Bang. The concept of the void returns in many myths and spiritual parables. From the womb to the waters of the ocean, the void symbolizes the prebirth state. The amorphous, uncrystallized nature of obsidian draws deep parallels to this state of being. As we cut away what doesn't serve us and look deep within to clear our shadow self, we become empty and radiant; we can then birth new possibilities by embracing the void.

If we look closely enough at the structure of volcanic glass we find that there are small clusters of molecules that exhibit short-range order. This means that the groupings of these molecules are in a precrystalline state—they are crystalline growth waiting to happen. A look at the larger picture reveals no orderly arrangement of crystal lattices throughout the matrix of obsidian, and this can look like chaos sweeping through the void. Obsidian empowers us to release our attachment to the mind and the ego and to step into this creative void. It is only possible to do so when we make room for that emptiness by not identifying with the mind.

The void represents the unknown, and our fears and aversion to uncertainty can hold us back from embracing it. However, when we accept vulnerability as strength-through-surrender, we see the truth behind the unknown: it is the womb in which our lives are carried to term, the blank slate on which we can paint the landscape of our lives. The silica-rich composition of obsidian amplifies this presence, and through its use we can attain a true connection to the here and now unlike ever before.

The only real growth and happiness occurs in the present moment. Everything we do is all about the now. If we are attached to the past or the future, we cannot have an authentic experience of stepping into the void. Because it calms mental energies, obsidian grounds our entire being in the present moment. We can use it to cut away the ego, to reflect what is beneath it, and to thereby enter the greatest mystery of all. This state of awareness is akin to embracing uncertainty, because the void is truly unknowable. The most basic fear that prevents us from stepping into vulnerability and claiming our light as our birthright is the fear of not being good enough.

Obsidian can appear to be a harsh teacher when we look deeply into who we really are, but this rock actually helps us understand self-compassion. By looking into the structure of obsidian we see that it isn't necessary for us to fit any mold. In a mineralogical sense, obsidian doesn't fit the mold either; it is considered a mineraloid, meaning "mineral-like," rather than a true mineral. This lack of status as a mineral doesn't prevent obsidian from being made, or from it continuing to be useful on our planet. While obsidian helps us bring the darkness into the light, it can't fix all of our problems, and that is just the point. Obsidian's real job is to show us that we are perfect exactly as we are. We do not need to be perfectly crystallized in order to achieve perfection. We can release our grip on expectations and accept imperfection as being enough.

The Fires of Rebirth

Let's face it: up to this point, working with obsidian has been hard work. It isn't an easy first stone on the path to self-actualization, but it is the first leg of our journey because it brings us into contact with the veil between the worlds and helps us cross over this partition into the realm of pure consciousness, the void. Volcanic glass is an igneous rock, so it is born of lava erupting from the underworld. Among indigenous cultures volcanoes are often considered to be portals to other realms. As a portal, the point of origin could be considered a threshold or liminal zone.

Liminal zones have long enthralled humankind. Countless sacred sites and other sacred spaces are found in such liminal zones—at volcanoes, on fault lines, on ley lines, near water, and in other natural places that have supernatural associations. These places are revered as doorways or portals between this plane of existence and the spiritual planes. Obsidian reminds us of its own connection to liminal zones, even when polished into a mirror, as mirrors of all sorts have been connected to liminal zones for millennia because they show us the in-between realm that lies in the shadows. This is why they are often used for scrying.

The threshold between the worlds is the place of the mystical. Shamanic practitioners often tread past the membrane that separates levels of reality, and the vision quest is a test of readiness for this shamanic path, whereby the spiritual aspirant takes his or her first step on the journey. Crossing over into the other plane of existence can be difficult, but obsidian guides us and grounds us as we endeavor to do so. Our first truly visionary experiences blaze the trail for deepening spiritual practices, and we can ask obsidian to guide and anchor us when we make our journeys.

Obsidian is brought into the world through powerful forces. The eruptions of volcanoes are horrifically destructive and amazingly beautiful in their display of primal creativity. Forests, towns, and anything else standing in the path of the lava's flow can be lost, yet out of the ashes of these igneous events new life grows in newly fertilized soil. Thus volcanic activity is both destructive and generative; it links together death and birth in a cycle of creativity. The volcano is the ultimate symbol for the cauldron of transformation. This fiery womb serves as the birthplace of the soul, as depicted in the myths regarding Pele. The cauldron of the goddess is the birthplace of our new selves as we step onto the spiritual path.

Fire is essential to the practice of alchemy, so the fiery origins of obsidian make it an excellent metaphor for alchemical transformation.

The word *igneous* denotes rocks and minerals produced from the cooling of magma. It is derived from the Latin word *ignis,* which means "fire." It is also the root word of *ignition.* Obsidian's connection to fire serves as a metaphor for initiating the fires of purification and transmutation. Working with obsidian ignites the process of inner alchemy, whereby we transform our base self into a more rarified form. Because of this, obsidian is an initiation stone. With obsidian in our toolbox, we can step into the void and claim the initiatory experience that awaits us there.

MEDITATION

STEPPING INTO THE VOID

For this meditation, any piece of obsidian will work, but find one that is a comfortable size. I prefer to use palm-sized stones. My favorite piece of obsidian for this work is a polished sphere. The size and shape of it are perfect to cradle in my hand, and the smooth surface gives me something into which I can stare in order to open my awareness and connect to the heart of the stone. Remember that setting your intention before beginning any meditation or visualization will bring better results. This meditation is meant to encourage you to embrace change and experience wonder in your life; however, you can tailor it to suit any purpose, from helping you to gather courage to connecting to your soul's purpose.

Begin by cleansing your stone, then grounding and centering yourself. Feel the weight of the stone in your hands gently pressing down on your palms. Feel your awareness as you connect to the earth and breathe deeply several times until relaxed. As you enter a state of relaxed awareness, stare at the obsidian in your hand and capture its image in your mind's eye. Then close your eyes and picture your consciousness contracting its awareness to a tiny point of light deep inside you. Breathe deeply and exhale this point of light into the stone. Visualize yourself being carried on your breath with that point of light. As it reaches the obsidian, your consciousness-as-light slides easily through the solid surface. Inside the obsidian, your surroundings are at first dark as midnight. You look around, but it is difficult to get your bearings. You are truly in the void; the blackness and blankness of it is all-encompassing. Breathe deeply and allow your subconscious mind to bring up images, thoughts, feelings. These will usually reflect states of uncertainty or fears that you may have. Many of these images may trigger feelings of anxiety or discomfort. Allow yourself to ask what it is about a given scenario that makes you feel uncertain. Send love to each thought or image and release it back into the void. Repeat until the state of anxiety has loosened its grip on you, and you can experience the beauty of the void without fear or discomfort.

While in the creative void, you may next focus on a goal that you wish to set for yourself. Formulate an image or statement that reflects your desire. Fill yourself with joy and gratitude as you picture the positive outcome of this scene, and then release it into the void. Thank the void and the obsidian, and slowly return your awareness back to your body.

OBSIDIAN IN CRYSTAL HEALING

One of the chief uses of obsidian is for grounding. It was introduced to many crystal healers in the 1980s as a tool for healing imbalances of the root chakra, which provides our connection to the earth and regulates some of our most basic survival needs. For this reason obsidian is a stone that often carries a kind of warning label; several prominent authors have pointed out that it is not for the faint of heart. This admonition has been dropped in recent years as the popularity of the stone has increased. It is likely that the evolution in consciousness has assisted in this readiness to work with obsidian. As more competent healers and authentic seekers add this volcanic stone to their toolboxes, the human condition is being gradually healed of its shadow side.

Obsidian is often recommended for conditions related to the physical manifestations of mental and emotional conditions, as well as for circulatory conditions and for overall safety and a sense of well-being.

Remember that obsidian, as a glass, is not a solid material in the strictest sense. Glass is subject to flowing like any other liquid, albeit only at temperatures high enough to melt it. When cooled, obsidian's molecules are suspended in their arrangements just as if they were still in motion, and this internal structure, or lack thereof, is what builds resonance with the body's circulatory system. For those who suffer from poor circulation, especially when it leads to painful conditions, try using obsidian to encourage a healthy flow of blood in your extremities.

By gently dissolving blockages and tightness in the body, obsidian is also used to help alleviate aches and pains. This relates to its use in supporting the circulatory system, as relaxing the walls of constricted vascular tissues reduces impediments to blood flow. Placed on zones of muscular tension, obsidian will slowly dissolve the knots and areas of soreness in the body. Its longstanding use as a prehistoric hunting implement has also made obsidian a traditional choice for healing wounds; some cultures even used obsidian as a preventive measure to ward off wounds, ensuring the safety and well-being of the person carrying or wearing obsidian.

Hearkening back to an age in which magic-makers employed sympathetic resonance,* where like attracts or cures like, obsidian's igneous birth is associated with igniting the processes of metabolism and digestion, since digestion is ruled by the element of fire. Place this stone at the solar plexus to encourage a healthy digestive system and to alleviate an upset stomach.

For the crystal therapist interested in remediating mental and emotional conditions, obsidian is an excellent catalyst for growth and for attaining wholeness. This dark gemstone can help a person overcome grief, break the grip of addictions, and rise above depression. It does this by reflecting back to us what the shadow self sees in these negative

---

*Sympathetic resonance is a phenomenon in which a passive vibrating body or field responds to external vibrations of similar or enharmonic frequency; an illustration of this phenomenon is when a violin string resonates after another string of the same note has been played.

cycles, so we can shed light on them and release or integrate them as necessary. Many times these obstacles can be crutches that we use to numb the pain and fear associated with being vulnerable; obsidian can help us find our inner strength by embracing our inner warrior.

Tackling fear, anxiety, and trauma is one of obsidian's best uses. These negative emotions are all interrelated, and they preclude the experience of unconditional love. Obsidian will help to gradually expand the consciousness of the user until he or she feels empowered to take a step into the unknown—the void—and accept uncertainty as a part of life. Additionally, obsidian reinforces the root chakra, which rules the sense of belonging. When we understand that we belong to the big picture and are firmly grounded in our lives, love and compassion make us feel buoyant enough to soar past the obstacles of worry and fear.

As a stone for spiritual healing, obsidian's key word is *illumination*. It serves to bring the darkness into the light such that we are able to look into our shadow self and flood it with unconditional love. Obsidian works by bridging the physical plane and the realm of the subconscious. It helps us develop a sense of inner freedom as we cross the threshold into the void. A truly shamanic stone, obsidian reinforces our support systems as we begin to feel comfortable dwelling in the liminal zones in life.

Obsidian shards, arrowheads, spearpoints, and polished wands or knives can be used to cut etheric cords and negative thought forms, foreign energies, and other attachments from the aura. To do so, cleanse and empower your obsidian and locate the area in question. Use a cutting motion to remove etheric cords; you may be guided to cut in one fell swoop or to saw back and forth depending on the nature of the energy at hand. To exorcise negative thought forms, imagine that the sharp edge of the obsidian is akin to a surgeon's scalpel. It can be used to cut away energies that do not belong in the aura, especially those that the client wants to release and has not been successful in doing so on her own. Always remember to seal the aura afterward. This can be accomplished by using an uplifting gemstone, such as clear quartz or selenite, and mentally projecting light or healing through the stone and into the void left by cutting with the obsidian. Afterward, smooth the aura with this stone, and visualize the energetic wound closing permanently.

As techniques of crystal healing have advanced, the uses of obsidian have also advanced. Nowadays, experienced therapists use varieties of obsidian for awakening the earth star chakra, located approximately one foot below the feet, thus deepening our connection to the earth. This volcanic mineraloid brings spirit into the material realm to more fully embody the true sense of self. It can help humankind ready itself for the changes at hand because of the rapid changes that resulted in its own formation. Obsidian is truly a powerful tool, and each of its varieties can be used for obtaining specific results.

Varieties of Obsidian

Apache Tears

These obsidian nodules are found in a soft matrix of perlite, which is another kind of volcanic glass. Perlite has a high water content and often forms from the hydration of obsidian during its initial formation. This in turn results in a softer host rock in which the Apache tears are formed. They are slowly weathered out of their matrix, and this is akin to being carried in a womb; even the higher water content of perlite is analogous to our watery, primordial birth. Because of this, Apache tears help us to explore our childhood, and they can help us release the tears we have held in check as a result of the conditioning we experienced during our formative years. Apache tears tend to be clearer than many other varieties of obsidian, and they can therefore help lend clarity to the process of sifting through our emotions, memories, and limiting beliefs. Use Apache tears during any time of loss, to anchor your aware-ness of grief in the physical body. They help to release repressed tears as well as to resolve the underlying issues surrounding them. Apache tears are ideal stones for anyone undergoing transition or loss.

Golden and Silver Sheen Obsidian

These two varieties of obsidian derive their velvety, iridescent appearance from inclusions of minute bubbles of gases or water as well as needlelike crystals of other minerals. These inclusions have a preferential orientation, allowing light to reflect off them when held only at certain angles. Sheen obsidians can appear dull and dark from one angle, and then they awaken with a glimmering, metallic light from another. This dual nature lends them to reconciling the duality experienced in life in the third dimension: life and death, light and dark, fear and love. Working with these stones can produce strong effects, and they are typically associated with visionary experiences, enhanced dreaming, or effective scrying. Obsidian can have iridescence of other colors, too, such as purple, brown, green, or blue, although these sheens are quite rare. Golden sheen obsidian tends to be more masculine, solar, and energizing, while silver sheen obsidian is often cooler, more introspective, feminine, and lunar in vibration. They pair nicely and can be used for insight into stunted spiritual growth or for transcending a plateau in the healing process.

Green Obsidian

Although many authorities do not recognize gem-quality colored obsidian as naturally occurring, there are indeed a few locations that produce such a stone. Transparent green obsidian has more of a heart focus than other members of the volcanic glass family, and its relative purity, due to lesser quantities of metallic elements, endows it with a loftier vibration as a whole. This gemlike natural glass activates the intelligence of our hearts, and it helps us to attain a level of transparency in all our endeavors. The brightly colored chartreuse obsidian, according to Katrina Raphaell, helps to rebuild "a positive self-image following a loss or tragedy" as well as to "burn the dross of insecurities."[12] It does this by breaking through the layers of scarcity consciousness that are conditioned into our psyches. Green obsidian is also recommended for removing and preventing energetic cords that attach to the heart center or to the emotional body.[13]

Mahogany Obsidian

The russet color found in mahogany obsidian, often dappled with and layered on darker colors, serves as the inspiration for its name. Mahogany obsidian has a much more physical focus than other members of the obsidian family. It is gently grounding, with a strengthening and toning effect, too. This formation of obsidian helps us develop a healthy body image and bolsters self-confidence by helping us see the beauty in our physical form. The color is due to the presence of iron oxides such as magnetite or hematite, and these minerals are both strongly grounding. Connecting with mahogany obsidian is at once grounding and refreshing, much like a walk through nature. It can be applied to the solar plexus for an energizing effect, as well as for healing repressed memories relating to body image. Carrying a piece can lend extra support and confidence to any situation, from a first date to a corporate presentation.

Rainbow Obsidian

Of all varieties of obsidian, rainbow obsidian often captures the eye's attention in ways that no other form of the stone can. When polished, this type of volcanic glass exhibits bands of iridescent colors—blue, green, purple, gold, and silver—against a black background. Each band is characterized by a distinct color due to a preferential orientation of microcrystals of mica and feldspar, although other minerals may also contribute to the rainbow effect. Both mica and feldspar can be iridescent, and in the formation of this obsidian they distribute as the lava slowly moves and then rapidly cools. Other minerals of varying degrees of density can also precipitate into bands of molten lava with degrees of viscosity.

Using rainbow obsidian opens the door to our hidden parts. It can heal anger and fear by facilitating the discovery of their cause and assisting us in finding the best way to move beyond them. Rainbow obsidian helps the mind to hone in on the root causes of disease and emotional patterns. It works by gradually resolving the issue layer by layer, just as its concentric bands reveal themselves. Rainbow obsidian helps us navigate the darkness in order to find the light in any situation. It bestows hope and encourages the first timid steps into the void.

Rainbow obsidian is best appreciated when polished. The act of polishing any kind of gemstone is the strategic stripping away of the host matrix, inclusions, and rough surfaces in order to reveal the inherent beauty of the rock or mineral. The lapidarist isn't adding anything to the stone to make it more beautiful; rather, she or he is only allowing the beauty that has always been there to be seen. Similarly, we must experience the discomfort of polishing our own hearts through surrender. Vulnerability is the state in which we surrender and become transparent. As we step aside and allow our dark corners to be filled with the light, the beauty already within us truly shines forth.

Snowflake Obsidian

Snowflake obsidian takes its name from the scattering of grayish spherules found against its black background. These spherules form as crystals of cristobalite, a high-temperature polymorph of quartz, begin to grow as radial aggregates inside the still-molten obsidian. Ultimately, the rock cooled too quickly for other minerals to crystallize as well. The pattern of these markings resembles snowflakes, and not surprisingly this particular member of the obsidian family tends to have a very active energy.

Movement and *illumination* are the key words I associate with this variety of obsidian. It can be used to help ignite a new direction, or it can add momentum to what is already in motion. Its effects are quite balancing, much like the balanced light and dark found in its structure. The crystals emerging from the void shine a metaphorical light into the dark areas of our beings. Because of this, snowflake obsidian can be used to locate sources of inspiration and hidden fears on the mental and emotional levels, as well as target pockets of infection in the physical body. Use snowflake obsidian when a new idea or the "eureka" moment of illumination is desired.

Related Stones

Let's take a look at some of obsidian's cousins. Each of these is also a glass, terrestrial or otherwise, and can be used for many of the same applications as obsidian. Some of these may be difficult to locate, so always ensure that you are purchasing from a trusted source when seeking new gemstones for your toolbox.

Tektite

Tektites are vitreous rocks that form as impactites—gravel-sized stones that are created by the force or heat of an impact. There are several theories regarding their exact formation, the most popular being the terrestrial theory—that tektites are the result of terrestrial material being thrust into the atmosphere during meteoric impacts. Other potential origin theories for these rocks point to the moon, suggesting that they consist of material that was ejected from the moon by major hydrogen-driven lunar volcanic eruptions and then drifted through space to later fall to Earth as tektites. Other authorities have even supposed that they may result from volcanism, human activity, comets, and natural fires. The most common variety of tektite is the indochinite tektite, which is a natural glass that appears black until held to the light. In thin slices it appears to be a greenish brown.

The name of these odd stones comes from the Greek *tēktós,* meaning "molten," which attests to their similarity to obsidian. Both mineraloids share similar compositions, and tektites were once thought to be an unusual formation of volcanic glass until their extraterrestrial origins were proposed. Tektites, which could be considered "space obsidian," marry the energies of Earth and the stars. They can expand consciousness and are frequently employed in enhancing the psychic senses or for encouraging contact with intelligences from other worlds. Tektites can anchor changes occurring in our spiritual bodies to our physical forms, and they often expedite the process of spiritual growth.

Moldavite

This is the most famous of the tektites. Moldavite is found mostly in the Czech Republic. It is a green, transparent tektite believed to have formed fifteen million years ago. It has been called the "grail stone," referring to the legend that the Holy Grail was carved from an emerald that fell from the sky.[14] Evidence of its use as a gemstone and as arrowheads extends back to Neolithic times.

Moldavite is a stone of transformation. Its energy is truly cosmic in scope, and it initiates swift and intense spiritual awakening. Moldavite can increase one's intuition, activate or stimulate the energy centers of the body, and detoxify each of the subtle bodies, purging them of unneeded patterns. Many people experience strong reactions to it, ranging from the "Moldavite flush," a reddening of the skin and warmer body temperature, to an all-out healing crisis. Moldavite expands awareness and unapologetically opens our eyes to our spiritual and emotional wounds. Working with moldavite is a great adjunct to using obsidian, as the two balance the influx of spiritual energy.

Libyan Desert Glass

Libyan desert glass (LDG) is perhaps one of my favorite natural glasses. The color is pale yellowy gold, sometimes leaning toward green, and it is found in the Great Sand Sea of the Sahara Desert. Its origin is likely meteoric, although it is not always classified as a tektite. Rather than being an impactite, LDG is generally regarded to be ejecta from the crash site of a meteor or a result of radiative melting from the heat generated by the meteor's impact. Dating tests have indicated that it formed 26 million years ago.

This particular glass is very pure silica, and it has one of the lowest water contents of any form of glass on Earth. It truly embodies golden light, and as such is a strongly empowering gemstone. LDG activates the strength of our will to its full potential, and this can yield excellent results for manifestation, especially with regard to money, employment, and confidence. This glassy gem helps you realize your full potential, both in the material and in the spiritual realms. King Tutankhamen was buried with a now-famous carving of LDG, which formed the centerpiece as an ornately carved scarab on a pectoral pendant. In ancient Egypt, this stone's regenerative properties were clearly known and used even in the afterlife. This stone truly embodies a sense of joy, and wearing it makes me feel as though I can accomplish anything. Incidentally, that is usually what happens when I do wear it.

Fulgurite

Fulgurite is natural glass formed when lightning strikes sand, soil, or rock. Fulgurite forms as delicate, hollow tubes in branching shapes. They are commonly found in Florida and Morocco. When lightning strikes, the temperature is actually hotter than the surface of the sun, which causes the silica in the sand to vaporize and expand rapidly. The cooling silica fuses quickly, and the result is a vitreous tube of natural glass.

Fulgurite is a powerful reminder that spiritual awakening is a spontaneous process; no matter how much preparation we undertake, we can never make enlightenment happen. Fulgurite helps show us that the separate, disparate pieces of ourselves must be integrated into wholeness as we grow spiritually, just as grains of sand are fused into glass. Fulgurite shows that the path to spirit is a path of emptiness: we cannot experience transformation unless we empty ourselves of our egos, expectations, and attachments. These hollow glass formations make excellent tools for communicating with the heavenly realms. Try holding them during meditation or whispering your prayers through a fulgurite to ensure that they will be heard and swiftly answered.

Andara Glass

I know that including a material such as this here might be controversial, but I cannot help but feel a great attraction to this enigmatic glass. There is no consensus about its genesis; it is likely that at least some of the deposits are man-made, while the Indonesian material is possibly of volcanic origin. True Andara glass only comes from a couple of deposits, including California and Indonesia, although similar materials have been found in Hawaii, Florida, and South Africa. The original source, however, is California, and theories about the origins of this glass are dubious at best. Andara is characterized by the range of colors in which it is found, including greens, pale blues, yellow, amber, reddish brown, and occasionally lavender and pink. Hues of clear, champagne, and seafoam green also exist. The material from Indonesia is mostly aquamarine in color, occasionally exhibiting patches of green, colorlessness, and gold; it sometimes contains inclusions of volcanic ash.

Andara is generally quite gemlike, and the pieces tend to seem candescent and luminous. While the California material was the first discovered, the variety from Indonesia is exceptionally beautiful, with a very pure energy to it. Andara glass is a spiritual accelerant. It tends to open the aspirant to deeper and more moving spiritual experiences. It is a tool for questioning, and working with it invariably leads to questions, for its origin is uncertain, its optical properties do not match those of other glasses, and it frequently changes color before one's eyes. Andara works to open your eyes to the wonder all around you. These noncrystals show us the inherent light of beauty and perfection in all things.

Working with Andara glass is a catalyzing experience. It is a potent vehicle of manifestation that requires a clear intent and fills your heart with pure trust. Whether it is natural or man-made, Andara glass calls us to evolution. Each call is unique and tailored to the individual working with it. This special glass initiates change through wonder. Open your heart when you work with this material, and expect magic to occur.

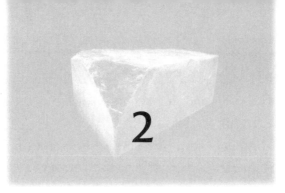

2

JADE

The Mask and the Immortals

Most precious gemstones' value can be measured by their color, clarity, and size, but some truly exceptional stones exist on another continuum altogether. Imagine a gem that has been prized by kings on virtually every continent, has started wars, and was believed to grant immortality. This stone is so precious that in the form of small river-tumbled pebbles it is worth its weight in gold, yet it can also be mined as boulders weighing thousands of pounds. The gem is jade, and it has been held in high esteem for millennia due to its color, durability, rarity, and the fine polish it takes in the hands of a skilled craftsman. To the Maya it was the stone of dreams; to the Chinese it was the stone of heaven.

The English word *jade* can be traced to the French *l'ejade* and the Latin *ilia,* meaning "flanks," "kidney area," and the Spanish *piedra de la hijada,* meaning "stone of the flank." When the Spaniards first encountered this green gem they learned that it was traditionally used to treat disorders of the kidneys, thereby healing pain in the flanks, or sides of patients' bodies, as well as prescribed for ameliorating colic and other conditions characterized by pain in the sides of the body. *Nephrite* is a term that was coined in the eighteenth century to describe the mineral first known as jade, and this term owes its provenance to the Greek word for *kidney*. Today, both varieties of jade are still employed for healing the kidneys in many traditions.

THE TWO JADES

Jade is actually comprised of two different materials: nephrite and jadeite, both metamorphic rocks that consist of different silicate materials. Though both materials have been used since prehistoric times for carvings, it has only been since the nineteenth century that what is known as jade was discovered to be two different minerals. Before looking into jade's connection with the mystery traditions, let's first look at the differences and similarities between the two species.

Nephrite: Classical Jade

Nephrite is the classical jade of China. It is actually an aggregate of two different minerals in the amphibole series, actinolite and tremolite. Both are monoclinic* minerals, and as a result of nephrite's metamorphic origin they blend together as interlocked, twisted fibers. Typically, nephrite is formed in regions that are subject to regional metamorphism, such as when tectonic activity yields mountains. These places, called "zones of orogeny," subject the parent rocks to low-grade pressure that gradually increases over eons; with greater pressure comes greater heat, and the end product is a gradually metamorphosed matrix of rocks. The interlocking fibers comprising nephrite are the source of its strength; they give the rock an irregular fracture and lend tenacity to the material, making it a durable choice for carving.

Nephrite can be found in many colors, depending on the mix of its two constituent minerals as well as the presence of accessory minerals and other trace elements. A predominance of white or gray is due

---

*In crystallography, the monoclinic crystal system is one of the seven lattice point groups. A crystal system is described by three vectors. In the monoclinic system, the crystal is described by vectors of unequal lengths.

to a larger amount of tremolite, while colors such as green, yellow, and brown are due to the higher iron content of actinolite.[1] Nephrite jade is commonly sourced from several different locations in China, where it is deposited by the flow of rivers and streams, though it is also mined in situ in places such as Kunlun, on the northern edge of the Tibetan Plateau.[2] Other important sources of nephrite include Canada (British Columbia), Australia, New Zealand, Taiwan, Poland, Italy, and Central Asia's Siberia; in the United States it is found in Alaska, Oregon, Washington, Wyoming, and California.[3]

Jade was given the name *yu,* written as the Chinese ideogram 玉, a term which now applies to all varieties of jade and is occasionally used to describe other jade-like minerals. Jade rose to fame among early Chinese cultures as it did in other locations worldwide due to its hardness and durability. As a material that withstood the wear of regular use, jade was favored over other stones because of its propensity to outlast other materials from which tools were fashioned that were not as hard. Nephrite's various colors were highly esteemed, although green appears to have been the most sought-after of all the hues of jade. As a relatively precious and extremely durable gem, nephrite jade evolved into a stone that was reserved for the aristocracy, the ruling class, and learned philosophers, and it was believed to be closely linked to the gods of abundance and the legendary immortals of Chinese mythology.

Carving jade became an art form that evolved during all the different Chinese dynasties. Jade was regarded as a status symbol as well as an auspicious gem that conferred longevity, good fortune, and a peaceful, virtuous life to its owner. Ritual implements continued to be manufactured from jade long after it became easier to make similar items from metal or other artistic mediums. The different Chinese dynasties carved jades that were said to be the color of "mutton fat" and "chicken bone."[4] Several naming conventions exist for describing the numerous shades of tomb jades, the artifacts that were buried with the dead that oxidized and became a new color. Above all other colors, the richest greens commanded the highest value. The dreamy nature of this stone seduced many merchants and emperors, and its status was elevated to that of stone of heaven—for it was believed it "had been hacked from a rainbow"[5]—a title it proudly wears even to the present.

Jadeite: Imperial Jade

The rarer, more precious variety of jade is jadeite. It has been given many names throughout the centuries, including *fei cui,* the Chinese name for the kingfisher, a bird that displays brilliant green feathers. Jadeite was relatively unknown to the ancient Chinese, although it was the jade referred to as the "stone of kings" that was used extensively in Central and South America. Jadeite, like nephrite, is also an admixture of minerals. This form of jade is a granular mass of interlocking pyroxene crystals, predominantly a silicate of sodium and aluminum, although other pyroxenes, such as acmite (a.k.a. aegirine) and diopside, may be present in varying amounts. This state of solid solution, in which varying components substitute for one another in the formation of rocks and minerals, is what accounts for the richness and variety of jadeite's color palette.

This type of jade is also generally found in areas of regional metamorphism, like its sister jade, nephrite. Rocks and their constituent minerals formed this way are subjected to high pressure and relatively low temperatures. Subduction zones, or areas in which one of the earth's tectonic plates is forced under another, as well as zones of orogeny, where mountains are formed from colliding tectonic plates, are ideal environments for the birth of jade. The resultant stone is necessarily resistant to erosion because of its fine-grained texture and gives jade its association with immortality.

Jadeite is often referred to as "imperial jade" because of its relative scarcity as well as its association with the Emperor Qianlong of the Chinese Qing Dynasty. Qianlong was held under the spell of this gorgeous greenstone, and he waged wars in order to source it from Burma

(Myanmar), where it is most abundant. Its rich, green color is due to the presence of chromium, and the granular structure of its monoclinic crystals grants a harder stone with a higher degree of translucence than nephrite jade. This propensity for allowing light to penetrate the surface of the gemstone gives jadeite a quality of candescence, in which it appears to be illuminated from within.

Jadeite, though rarer than nephrite and sourced much later in China's lapidary history, was actually the first gem to be named "jade" among Europeans. When the Spanish conquistadores returned from exploring the Americas, they brought with them the curious *piedra de hijada,* which was so highly prized among the Maya. The priestly class of Mesoamerican cultures regarded jade as a dream stone because it was believed to connect them to the spiritual world beyond our own. As with the Chinese, the Maya also interred the deceased with jade in order to help them reach the pinnacle of the afterlife. To the Maya, jade ensured safe passage and guided the soul of the departed through eternity. For these reasons, jadeite was more highly prized than any other precious stone, more coveted than gold among the Olmec, Maya, and other Mesoamerican peoples.

Jadeite can be found in other regions, too. Central Japan is home to one of the world's few sources of this gemstone, and while white jade is the most common type found there, it is also found in lively greens, black, blue, and violet shades.[6] The Japanese used jade as a sacred stone and carved it into talismans like the magatama, commalike or hook-shaped beads that originated in prehistoric Japan. It is possible that these mysterious stones, which at one time were quite prolific, are descended from the shape of animals' teeth or claws.[7] These enigmatic shapes were similarly used in Korea, especially as ornaments for royalty such as crowns. The magatama more than likely were used to signify authority, and one is even regarded as part of the three sacred relics of the Imperial Regalia of Japan.[8]

In India, jadeite was used in Vedic astrology, while it served as a talisman of the planet Mercury in the ayurvedic tradition, where it was generally used as a substitute for emerald.[9] In other astrological systems, jade of any type is frequently associated with Venus, the planet that rules love and romance.

Comparing Nephrite and Jadeite

Both of these forms of jade are comprised of minute crystals of their constituent minerals, and each belongs to the monoclinic crystal system. Nephrite owes its texture and toughness to the interwoven masses of fibrous crystals of actinolite and tremolite. This makes it more resistant to breaking than jadeite, despite jadeite's lower hardness. Jadeite's composition is granular, and the interlocking grains of pyroxene minerals make it denser and harder than nephrite; it is, in fact, harder than steel. This difference in structural composition gives each form of jade a slightly different affinity for healing. The compositions of each variety of jade prevent it from achieving transparency. Though typically opaque, the finest pieces may be translucent at best, with jadeite's granular structure permitting more light to penetrate. Because of this, jadeite is the more luminous of the two varieties of jade.

These variations in composition and structure account for differences in the energies contained in jade. Generally, nephrite's fibrous crystals encourage a flow of energy. This translates to both the physical and the nonphysical aspects of our lives, from the free-flowing of the life force, or chi, to the healthy flow of liquids in the eliminatory and circulatory systems. Nephrite tends to feel more electric, almost as though it is in motion. On the other hand, the minute, compacted grains of jadeite are very stabilizing. They extend a grounding and anchoring influence to the body, mind, and spirit. This is felt in terms of physical safety and peace of mind. Both gemstones contain a number of common elements among their constituents. For this reason, both nephrite and jadeite have a great number of spiritual properties in common.

AN OVERVIEW OF JADE'S SYMBOLISM

It is beyond the scope of this work to document every category of artifact commonly carved from jade, or to record every known use among the dozens of cultures to have known jade intimately. The fact is that jade meant a lot of different things to a lot of different people. Because of this, I have worked to distill the essence of the archetypes of jade as they are relevant within the context of other stones found in this book. In light of this, before moving on to the major archetypes, jade deserves an overview of its most common associations.

Owing largely to its color and fineness, jade stands out among other rocks. The lush and vibrant greens and earthy tones have long brought associations of new life and growth to mind. Among the Olmec, blue shades of jadeite linked this stone to the maize deity as their corn was blue in color. The primary source of sustenance for the Olmec, corn was the symbolic life force. Similarly, their successors, the Maya, revered green jade; its prized imperial color reminded them of fertile plant growth and the greenish waters of sacred springs. Jade is the color of nature and was created by the gods to solidify the association with life. It conferred fertility in many cultures, and jade of all varieties nourished its wearer, both in this life and beyond.

In the South Pacific, the Maori of New Zealand knew jade, as well as other greenstones, as *pounamu*. This "greenstone" was often carved into waves, fern spirals, and fierce ancestral spirits known as *hei-tiki*. Pounamu represented not only life and nature but also power. The tribal leaders of the Maori carried a type of club called a *mere*, which served as much as a symbol of strength as an effective weapon in battle. In fact, jade represents sovereignty in virtually every culture that has had access to it, and it often was fashioned into clubs, scepters, celts (prehistoric stones shaped like a chisel or axe head), and other handheld implements to denote the authority of whoever should carry them.

Jade is a stone of heavenly power even in modern China. Among ancient people of the Far East it developed the reputation of being a peaceful stone of great virtue, one associated with heaven and good fortune. Among archeological remains unearthed in Asia, virtually every manner of jade has been discovered. Jade was so universally respected and treasured that even the most common of household implements have been made from it at one time or another. The Chinese of many dynasties shaped jade into ornaments, jewelry, ceremonial implements, and objects of great beauty. Tomb jades abound in archeological digs because of the widespread belief in jade's immortal qualities. It has been thought to confer longevity and immortality to its wearers, and it has been found in gravesites across China in the form of funerary masks, votive offerings, and even entire suits. The custom of placing jade into the mouths of the dead was a routine practice not only in several Asian cultures but also in Mesoamerica and Egypt.[10]

Jade has been elevated to one of the most prized gemstones, and has been frequently reserved for the aristocratic classes. This stone has even served as currency in several places around the world, and its associations with wealth and good fortune are among its best-known attributes today. Across the planet, polished bangles, carved pendants, and rounded beads of jade grace the bodies of millions of people who seek to harness jade's many qualities to improve their lives.

JADE AS AN ARCHETYPE: THE MASK

Masks evoke an air of mystery. They are both elusive and revelatory, disfiguring and transfiguring. To don a mask is to become the subject of the mask, and for that reason they have long been associated with shamanic rites and the earliest mystery school teachings. They are primal symbols of the unknowable, and the use of masks persists in traditions both spiritual and profane even today. The earliest depictions of personified deities tend to be masked, schematized figures. The extensive work of pioneering archeologist Marija Gimbutas recreates the role of religious thought and practice in the Stone Age through the observation of arts and crafts as found in the archeological remains of early societies.[11] Gimbutas's research shows that early human representations of the divine were nearly always masked because the true nature of Source is beyond mortal comprehension.

Masks serve practical purposes, too, for they are protective and may prevent harm. Wearing a mask keeps away debris and averts injury. The mask hides the wearer's identity and allows him or her to assume a new one. The human psyche has adopted the habit of assuming masks throughout a person's lifetime. These personas, which owe their very name to the Greek word for mask, are a mental and emotional identity meant to hide fears and doubts as well as to ward off the most minuscule opportunity for shame.

Masks carved from jade are a prominent motif among both Eastern and New World jade cultures. Funerary masks carved from jade were intended to bestow eternal life to their wearers and assuage the effects of decomposition of the physical body after death.[12] The kings of the Olmec and Maya peoples were buried with elaborate masks, sometimes carved from solid pieces of jade and sometimes from mosaics of the stone. Similar masks are pervasive in Chinese burials, and entire suits of jade tiles strung together have even been disinterred. These tomb jades exist not just because of jade's connotation of physical immortality; jade is regarded as a nurturing stone, one that is meant to feed the soul of the deceased for eternity. Funerary masks in Mesoamerica often had celts of jade attached to them, meant to represent the breath of the wearer. Not unlike the carvings placed inside the mouths of the dead, these artifacts were intended to feed the spirit of those who cross into the next life by providing spiritual breath and sustenance to their nonphysical selves.

Jade's connotation of immortality arises not only from its exceptional beauty and virtue, but also from its hardness and tenacity. While these qualities make it a difficult stone to carve, jade withstands the erosive nature of time itself. It confers a symbolic immortality to the carver, whose art lives on forever, as well as to the bearer of the jade. In an ancient act of utilizing the power of sympathetic resonance, to display a substance that never decays can guard against death and decomposition. Jade is physically harder than steel, and so it was among the most long-lasting of any carving medium available.

Stripping Away the Ego

Masks are hollow, empty, and illusory. We wear masks in our day-to-day life because we are told from an early age to "put on a brave face" or to behave a certain way in specific situations. Over time, the behaviors we adopt to hide our thoughts, hopes, and fears become metaphorical masks that we oftentimes take to the grave. These masks are generally limiting because we begin to identify with them, rather than use them as mere tools.

Masks hide our fear of the unknown as well as the inherent fear of disconnection. But as we wear them, we actually become a living paradox by guarding our authentic selves from ever being known and making true connections. The original purpose of the mask was to endow the faceless, formless, and unknowable creative force of the universe with a personified and identifiable form. Nowadays we attire ourselves with mental masks to make ourselves unknown; this is a breeding ground for insecurity and psychosis.

The true message of the jade mask is one that is shared with the jade skull carvings of the Americas, Mongolia, and China. The majority of these jade skulls are hollow, not unlike masks, and they differ from skulls carved from other stones and from crystal (such as the crystal skulls described in chapter 6). Ultimately, the skull, like the mask, asks us to strip away false pretenses and attachments. We release our concerns and fears about our form and identity so we can receive from the heavens and continue to grow spiritually. This belies the axiom that "you only keep what you give away," because the laws governing the spiritual plane are inverse to those ruling physical reality. By releasing, we make room to receive; this is what makes jade such an effective stone for abundance and material wealth.

The jade mask requires you to be brutally honest with yourself.

Your true self lies behind your persona, behind your ego, behind your fear. It exists outside of the temporary, physical body that is destined to decay. We can learn to replace the psychological mask with the jade mask, and when we do it marks the death of the ego and the death of fear in favor of the immortal spiritual self. Jade invites you to find the masks you wear and to cease identifying with them. Become empty, like the mask itself. This only takes place when you accept the nature of emptiness. When you peel away the masks of ego and identity, all that remains is the cosmic void within, and this void is the space where God dwells.

If obsidian can show us the void so that we can enter it, jade shows us where the void dwells so it may enter us. The mask, hollow and cold, is the empty vessel; it is the blank slate and the beginner's mind. The jade mask is our guide to pouring out our attachments so that the divine may fill us with peace. What we find within the inner void is truly the secret to immortality.

MEDITATION

REMOVING THE MASK

This meditation is best undertaken after becoming comfortable with the exercises in the previous chapter. Obsidian entrains the strength and vision necessary to move further into spiritual practice and begin peeling away the ego. Jade is a gentle teacher, but it has unwavering strength. If this meditation begins to show any signs of discomfort, shift your focus onto jade's stabilizing, tranquil frequency until the sensation passes.

Select a smooth piece of jade, either rough or polished. Lie comfortably with the stone on the brow, or third-eye, chakra. Visualize the stone growing in diameter until it covers your entire face, like a mask. As you breathe, imagine exhaling the ego and all of its machinations into the jade mask. Do this several times until it feels as if the mask has grown heavy and saturated.

Next, reach up and take hold of the stone. Gently lift it off your forehead, and as you do so, envision that you are slowly peeling off your mask of jade, along with all the ego's attachments, expectations, feelings of entitlement, and fears. When the mask is entirely removed, allow the image of the mask to dissipate into the ethers, as it is transmuted by the universe.

Next, place the jade on your heart center, in the center of the sternum, and allow it to begin to fill your newly emptied being with pure peace. When you have reached a point of fullness, permit the essence of peace to overflow and feed the earth and your surroundings. When you are complete, breathe deeply and gently, and open your eyes.

JADE AS AN ARCHETYPE: THE GUARDIAN

Myths of supernatural guardians permeate human history, and jade is not immune to consorting with these immortal beings. Motifs of dragons, feathered serpents, gods and goddesses, and ancestral protectors populate the legends of the stone of heaven. In art, these beings form universal motifs. They are the protectors and guardians of the spiritual seeker, and they serve as teachers and guides along the path.

Each of the supernatural guardians depicted in jade represents the natural forces and the essence of the immortals. Jade may have been chosen to depict these mythical creatures because of its longstanding connection to the natural world and the world of the gods and goddesses. As mentioned earlier, the colors in which jade minerals are found provide links to life itself, and life is a gift from the powers of creation. When coupled with this gemstone's ability to survive into eternity, it becomes the perfect medium for sculpting the immortal guardians.

The Jade Dragon

One jade image common in different cultures throughout the eons is that of the dragon. In China, while the manner in which dragons have been depicted in jade has changed from dynasty to dynasty, they are an omnipresent image in Chinese myth and history. The earliest jade dragons date back to the Hongshan Dynasty, around 4700 BCE. These early carvings may well be China's first representations of dragons in any medium. Across the expanse of millennia, dragons evolved from the simple, C-shaped figures of the Hongshan carvers, called *zhulong,* or "pig dragons," to the elaborate image of the Chinese dragon that one sees today.

The jade dragons of Chinese dynasties include zhulong, chimera-like dragons, and the feral-looking *tao-tie,* a masklike motif common to the Liangzhu Dynasty. These fierce, immortal creatures are guardians of the celestial kingdoms of Chinese culture. Because of jade's funerary associations, carvings of jade dragons traditionally accompanied other mortuary goods; these dragons were believed to have been a means for the deceased to travel to heaven. Both funereal and celestial locations can be considered liminal zones, thereby connecting jade to the threshold of the cosmic void, represented by obsidian.

Dragons in Chinese myth are supernatural beings that rule the phenomena of nature. They are known to bring rain, control thunder, dwell in springs and waterfalls, and guard the heavens. Dragons came to be associated with the emperor and other nobility, and a Chinese expression even describes the people of China as the "Descendants of the Dragon."[13]

On the opposite side of the globe, another draconic jade can be encountered—the Feathered Serpent, symbol of the Aztec god Quetzalcoatl. Quetzalcoatl is a deity whose worship spanned several Mesoamerican cultures. His attributes included dominion over death and resurrection; the morning star, Venus; and fertility. Two of his greatest gifts to humankind are calendars and maize. To the Maya he is known as the Feathered (or Plumed) Serpent, Kukulkan. At the temple of Chichen Itza at El Castillo there stands a special representation of him, a "life-sized jaguar with open jaws. Affixed to his frame were seventy-two discs of polished jade, each apple-green, a curious application of precious *chalchihuitl* [jade] to the fearsome cult-beast."[14] The Feathered Serpent acts as a guardian of the liminal space between life and death and is often associated with the wind. This personification of natural phenomena like the wind is not unlike that of the Chinese dragons, and it connects the guardian archetype to the breath of life.

The archetypal jade dragons are given dominion over the natural world. Their affinity with elemental energy and the control of weather, water, and life makes them personifications of nature itself. Jade, whose colors echo the blues of water and the greens of plant life, shares this connection to nature through sympathetic resonance. This link is the source of jade's association with abundance and fertility, and consciously working with jade provides the opportunity to experience this on all levels, from a fertile garden to a ripening of inspiration or sprouting seeds of spiritual understanding. Jade reminds us that the spiritual path starts from our physical, natural existence and grows toward the heavens, just as maize and other plants point their growth toward the light of the sun.

Other Guardian Figures in Jade

As noted above, in Mesoamerican cultures carvings of jade figurines often accompanied the dead to their final resting place. These supernatural beings included the corn maiden, were-jaguars, and numerous birdlike creatures. While the purpose and symbolism of each of these figures may be hard to determine individually, they all resonate to the archetype of the guardian. Rather than being a symbol of immortality like the jade mask or the jade placed in the mouth of the deceased person, the jade guardians are the guides, protectors, and teachers necessary to complete the shaman's journey to nonordinary reality.

Skilled Maori carvers in New Zealand craft elaborate hei-tiki, another form of ancestral guardian, from greenstone. "The hei-tiki is the most important jade artifact created by the Maoris . . . Also made of jade were smaller ornaments called *peka-peka,* some in the shapes of fishes, others like serpents."[15] The hei-tiki is a humanlike being, with a tilted head bearing large eyes; they often have webbed fingers and toes and grimacing, beaklike mouths. These talismans are named after

Tiki, the "first man," and therefore represent the line of ancestors of the wearer's bearer.[16] The hei-tiki was usually buried with its owner until later being exhumed by his successor. The power inherent in this style of carving was believed to be in proportion to the number of generations of owners.

Each type of jade guardian has a supernatural countenance, and most are depictions of immortals of one form or another, which is both a nod to jade's link to eternity as well as to the nature and function of the guardians themselves. The guardians are the helpers and teachers on the spiritual path. Jade resonates a peaceful frequency that attunes one to the natural and celestial realms; it is the receiver-transmitter for the spiritual guides and helpers who facilitate access to other planes of consciousness.

MEDITATION

MEETING YOUR GUARDIAN DRAGON

Each member of the human race incarnates with a complete set of spiritual guides, teachers, and way-showers, each of whom is ready and willing to lend a helping hand if only we learn to ask. In this meditation, jade will serve as a link to the realm in which the guardian archetype dwells. Choose a piece of jade that is comfortable for you, one that has a personality. For this meditation I have chosen a small carving of a dragon made from greenish jadeite. Although this exercise focuses on draconic guides, feel free to connect to any of your spiritual helpers and teachers by substituting the words that feel most comfortable.

Hold your jade comfortably in whichever hand you prefer. You may sit or lie, with closed eyes, as you allow your attention to center around the weight and texture of the stone in your hand. Allow your awareness of all else to slowly fade away until the stone is all that fills your focus. Imagine the stone in your hand is growing heavier; it seems to be moving into the earth, and it pulls you with it. Deeper and deeper you sink, until you enter a cavern within the body of the Earth Mother.

Within this sacred chamber your guardian dragon awaits. Bow

with reverence and introduce yourself to the dragon. Await his or her greeting, then begin a conversation. You are welcome to ask anything of your guardian. He or she can accompany you on your spiritual journey if invited, and this dragon can be a powerful ally in ascending to the next level of your growth.

When you have completed your first visit, thank the dragon for his or her time and offer the creature a symbolic gift of jade. Ask your dragon to return you to your body on the earth plane. When your consciousness arrives, breathe deeply and gradually return your awareness to the room. Repeat this meditation as often as you like when you are first getting to know this guide; after establishing good rapport, you can call on your dragon for assistance in all matters.

Jade in the Dreamtime

Jade acts as a guardian of the subconscious mind. Many cultures associate jade with the realm of dreams, and it has rightly earned the moniker "dream stone."[17] Jade is revered worldwide, even today, for the deep peace that can be felt when wearing this gemstone. It helps to relax the mind and acts a general tonic for the wellness of the physical body. Because it puts its wearer at ease and provides more restful sleep while averting nightmares, jade is one of the premier stones for accessing the dreamtime, a term that refers to different states of nonordinary reality, including shamanic journeying.[18]

The role of the shaman is to learn the language of the spiritual world and bring it back to benefit others. After honing one's courage and inner vision, as the archetypes of obsidian teach us, jade helps us further in accessing other realms of existence. "Jade is a stone of great wisdom . . . the most powerful stone of the dream state on earth, and initiates mastery on that level of self."[19] While you may first be drawn to use it for its peaceful influence, "you may find that it will help you in other-dimensional travels."[20]

Dreaming is a state of consciousness in which we can tap into eternity. During the dream state, the causal, or karmic, body is most active. Because of this, jade helps us experience time outside of the way it runs in ordinary reality. Jade provides the window through which we can meet our spiritual guardians and guides, listen to the voices of our ancestors, and even heal past lifetimes in order to resolve the karma attached to them. Jade helps rarefy our spirit through this resolution of karma such that we can come closer to achieving our first step into the celestial realms.

Jade permits access to the world of dreams because it is in this imaginal realm that dragons still roam. The guardian archetype makes itself known best when ordinary, waking consciousness is peeled away to reveal nonordinary reality. Jade is able to provide discipline in practicing these travels, just as discipline is required to cut and polish this harder-than-steel gem. Polishing jade "takes the scratches that have been made in the course of carving and grinding and gradually replaces them with finer and finer scratches until they're no longer visible to the human eye. The key word is *gradually*. Whereas softer stones, such as marble, take a polish relatively quickly, jade, thanks to its great density, must be coaxed to a luster."[21] We are told that jade's effects are slow, just like the process of polishing, and that it can "help detach from the emotions involved [in dream work] so that you can see more clearly."[22]

With patience and practice, the warrior who has learned courage and strength through surrender by means of the teachings of obsidian can identify a need to cultivate a relationship with the guardians and teachers of the jade archetype. Through meditation, dream work, and an open heart, jade helps us tap into the power and wisdom that these ancient guardians of liminal zones are willing to teach. The dragons and other immortal beings can be viewed as archetypal teachers and friends on the "road of trials" encountered on the hero's journey, as described by Joseph Campbell. These teachers and guardians walk the threshold of our world and the celestial realms; they are the intermediaries between the earthly and heavenly kingdoms.

Countless vessels and containers worked in fine jades are found in many parts of the world. These bowls, cups, and other containers represent a barrier or liminal space; a jade bowl, for instance, is a membrane that separates that which is within it from the world around it. These vessels form a symbolic barrier between the physical world and the non-physical world. Jade artifacts, especially those representative of physical health and fertility, are typically found in liminal zones such as tombs and bodies of water, because jade is the archetypal intermediary. While it does not belong wholly to the plane of the gods, it is also not entirely of a dense and earthy vibration.

As the archetype of the guardian, jade can be our greatest teacher. Obsidian helps us to answer the call to the spiritual path, but along the way it is inevitable that help is needed. Jade steps in to help us strip away our persona and seek guidance from the root of our true identity. This stone is the "sage of the gemstone world," and it can impart serenity through wisdom on "how to live in harmony with the laws of nature and the laws of spirit."[23] Through meeting your guides and teachers, jade reveals the path that bridges heaven and earth.

MEDITATION

DREAMING WITH JADE

As a dream stone, jade makes an excellent ally in exploring other levels of consciousness. For this exercise, choose a familiar piece of jade that is comfortable to hold at night or to keep underneath your pillow; polished or tumbled stones may work best. Keeping a pad and pen at hand makes it easy to record your experiences upon awakening in order to chronicle your adventures with jade.

Before falling asleep, hold your piece of jade in whichever hand is most comfortable. Bring the stone to your third-eye chakra and ask that jade open the gateway to the dreamtime to help you on your spiritual path. If you have a specific goal or intention, such as healing a particular condition, releasing a mental or emotional pattern, or meeting with your guides, state this goal in your dialogue with the energy of the gemstone. Once you have stated your intention, remove the stone from your forehead and either place it under your pillow or hold it in your palm throughout the night; don't worry if you let go of it while sleeping.

Imagine breathing in the energy of jade as you fall asleep. More than likely, your dreams will be especially vivid. Whenever you awaken, scribble down the elements of your dreams for later analysis. Look for repeating symbols or events over a longer course of time. Dreaming with jade can be a great way to reveal answers that other forms of divination and journeying may not otherwise provide.

JADE AS AN ARCHETYPE: THE GATEWAY TO HEAVEN

For centuries Chinese philosophers extolled the virtues of the stone of heaven. Jade is a powerful ally on the unfolding path of spiritual awakening because it guides us toward our goal of realizing our potential as heavenly beings incarnate in earthly bodies. The archetypes explored up to this point have only readied the seeker for reaching the gateway to the celestial realms, the final archetype we will explore in this chapter. The mask hides the doorway; it reminds one to look within rather than without for entry into higher states of being. The jade guardian watches over the doorway. The dragon guides those who are ready and will devour those who are not.

Jadeite and nephrite have been highly esteemed by the priestly and noble classes since the times of the ancients. It was a stone relegated to the educated and wealthy echelons of society because of its power to catalyze the process of rising up. Buried with the dead, jade helped the souls of the deceased rise up and stripped away those parts of their identities that could weigh them down. The stone of heaven is celestial in its own right, despite its dense, earthy vibration; this association comes not from being heavenly in and of itself, but because of the virtue and peace it evokes from within, which grants passage to heaven.

A number of carvings of jade allude to its role as the gateway, although the precise use of these carvings has been forgotten over millennia. In China, ceremonial jades played a significant role in ritual in the imperial court. Of these, two of the most iconic and enigmatic carvings are the *cong* (pronounced *tsong*) and the *bi* (pronounced *bee*). The cong is a tube with a circular inner section and squarish outer section. The outer surface is divided vertically or horizontally such that the whole defines a hollow cylinder embedded in a partial rectangular block. Examples range from several inches to more than a foot in length. Many times the squared edges of the cong are embellished with stylized faces, not unlike the feral countenances of the tao-tie mask. The bi, in contrast, is a round, flat disc with an open center. In its simplest form it is unadorned, although the bi can be very elaborate, with several discs stacked within one another, sometimes bordered by dragons and other mythical creatures.

The bi and cong are considered ceremonial jades by today's scholars, for they "designate jades used for imperial ceremonies."[24] These symbolic tools were generally used in groups of six, with four jade plaques used to represent the four directions. The bi and the cong completed the group, representing respectively heaven and earth. Jade has long been associated with the four directions in other parts of the world; in Mesoamerica, similar uses of jade have been unearthed.

Both of these ancient Chinese artifacts, the bi and the cong, typify the nature of the gateway to heaven. These objects are painstakingly polished and left with hollow cores. Jade serves as the way-shower on the path to heaven, teaching us to release what weighs down one's spirit in order to become lighter, freer. Thus the gradual process of polishing jade is a metaphor for the effects that jade's virtues have on our spiritual progress.

The Stone of Many Virtues

Much has been written describing the virtues that jade embodies. The Chinese imperial court coveted it in order to harness the peaceful virtue imbued in it. Among the philosophers of China, jade was emblematic of the Confucian and Taoist ideals, and Confucius spoke of its harmony, saying,

Wise men have seen in jade all the different virtues. It is soft, smooth, and shining—like kindness; it is hard, fine, and strong—like intelligence; its edges seem sharp, but do not cut[—]like justice; it hangs down to the ground—like humility; when struck, it gives a ringing sound—like music; the stains in it which are not hidden, and which add to its beauty—are like truthfulness; its brightness is like heaven, and its fine substance (born of the mountains and water) is like the earth.[25]

Jade, as the stone of heaven, was believed by the Chinese as well as the ancient Mesoamericans to confer the sovereignty of the heavens on those who wore it. The emperor of China possessed one of the world's finest collections of jades, from ceremonial jades to royal scepters. The use of these ritual objects in rites of public worship was to maintain harmony between heaven and earth. The emperor, known as the "Son of Heaven," served not only as the political leader of the people of China but also as their spiritual leader. His example in embodying the heavenly virtues aided his role in mediating between the spiritual and material planes. For this reason it is not surprising that the Chinese palace was littered with jade. Ultimately, jade's associations with fertility and wealth likely stemmed from its ability to connect with and serve the Source more mindfully.

The poet Maya Angelou states that of all the virtues, courage is the most important, for it enables the practice of all other virtues. Courage itself is derived from the French word *coeur,* "heart." Therefore, to be courageous is not necessarily to master bravado and fearlessness; rather, it is engaging in your path with your full heart. Jade has long been extolled as being a tranquil, heart-healing stone, and many modern texts on crystal healing associate its soft green color with the energy of the heart center. Jade truly helps to open the heart and apply the virtues contained therein to any situation.

Being virtuous is not an easy task. It takes practice, patience, and a certain amount of mental mastery to relinquish the self-judgment that inevitably follows when one falls short. This discipline is difficult to come by, but one can attain it with the help of jade. A polished piece of jade has undergone rigorous scraping, scratching, and buffing to refine its surface until it appears to glow. Spiritual practice is similar—the application of virtue to one's actions and thoughts will gradually refine and polish one's heart.

If obsidian, which is relatively brittle and somewhat soft for a gemstone, teaches us that we can attain progress on the spiritual path by allowing life to splinter us, break us open, and gently polish the mirror of our heart, then jade confers the secret of taking this process of rarefaction further. Jade lacks good cleavage, and its fracture is uneven and unyielding. Rather than cutting and polishing it like a transparent gem, it must be slowly abraded, which is painstaking work. Jade's toughness teaches us the discipline and integrity necessary to fashion our own roughness into a gemstone, thereby growing toward enlightenment. Ultimately, jade inspires the persistence and resiliency that are required for reaching a spiritual breakthrough. Through the constant polishing of our virtues, we have enough raw material to transform our lives into a "house full of jade, in which only the enlightened may enter" on the path to heaven.[26]

Rising to Heaven

Jade of any variety is prized for its toughness, texture, and density. The stone of heaven is a geological marvel, especially the rarer, precious variety, jadeite. Although known as a stone inviting deep peace, immortality, and good health due to its heavenly vibrations, the formation and composition of jade is anything but light and celestial. One of the determining characteristics of jade is its relatively high specific gravity, which is a measurement of its density. Most dense stones have a tendency to connect us to the earth, energetically speaking. The grounding qualities of jade, owing to its density and composition, certainly account for the profound peace and well-being felt when working with jade, but this leaves the heavenly connection in question.

Jade of either variety is formed by metamorphic activity. Metamorphic rocks are those that are formed as other rocks undergo changes due to shifts in temperature and pressure, such as during the collision of tectonic plates and the formation of mountains. As temperature and pressure rises, certain mineral constituents of rocks liquefy and rearrange themselves into new minerals. Metamorphic rocks invite the same idea of metamorphosis in our own lives; as we experience pressure from inner or outer resources, we can recrystallize and claim greater levels of strength and organization than we have ever known.

In particular, jadeite occurs in subduction zones, where one tectonic plate is forced below another where they meet. Oceanic plates are generally formed from an upper layer of the dense rock basalt. When the plates are subducted below a continent, the pressure and temperature rises, while "pressure forces some of the water out of the subducting plate, working like rollers of an old-time washing machine. Since some of the major components of jade—sodium, aluminum, and silicon—are all relatively soluble, they dissolve out of the metamorphosing basalt and are carried away and introduced into the overlying plate."[27] These components are packed together tightly, thereby granting jade its characteristic density.

Jadeite is seldom found alone; when prospecting one of the telltale signs that jadeite may be present is the presence of serpentine, a lighter, softer mineral species. Serpentine rocks, or serpentinite, form during the subduction process as parent rocks are exposed to seawater. It becomes the vehicle for jadeite to make its way to the surface. Jade, if left in its womb, will not remain stable, so it must quickly rise along faults in order to reach a stable environment. "The jade is embedded in the serpentinite like raisins in a pudding, and though jade is dense, the serpentinite is relatively lightweight; as the lighter rock is buoyed upward, the jade rides along with it."[28] All of these factors make it a very rare occurrence for jadeite to form at all, let alone reach its final destination, where we can find it and work with it.

The association of jadeite and its carrier stone of serpentine teaches us to take advantage of our environment. Today, jade is often worn or carried as a talisman for good fortune; it is this good fortune that jade recognizes in its friend, serpentine. If the two did not form together, jade would not exist at all, and if the timing of the two coming together does not play out just so, jade is lost before it ever can be found. Jade's energy stabilizes our entire being, especially the nonphysical body, and it keeps everything synchronized to the rhythm of the universe. This is how jade's presence in our lives seems to afford us better luck and fortune; we learn to live in the moment more and more by embracing and living in a peaceful, connected state.

The rise toward heaven that precious jade must undergo teaches us that our own ascent begins when we feel dragged under by the circumstances in our lives. Compassion, forgiveness, and surrender are too often only born in cases when one feels lost, with nowhere left to turn but to the Source. The stone of heaven helps us rise to a heavenly state of mind when we ask to be carried there by the guardians of heaven. The dragons, ancestors, and other immortal protector archetypes are always willing to take our hand and guide us upward.

Artifacts carved from jade commonly depict images and symbols associated with bridging heaven and earth. Clouds, birds, dragons, and even the wind are motifs that span virtually every greenstone-carving culture on Earth. These portrayals of beings that move from the earth into the skies symbolize the upward movement that jade makes. It is not a stone of lofty vibration that shines heavenly light down into us; instead, it is a dense earth stone that illustrates how terrestrial life in the material plane aspires to returning to heaven. Engravings of wind, breath, and clouds, in both the Old World and the New, inspire us so that the very breath of life entering us should uplift the human spirit, moving it toward the realm of the gods.

The rising, against all odds, of such a dense stone to the surface of the earth reminds us that no matter where we are in life, we too can rise up and out of our present circumstances. Jade may be a stone that is connected to more avenues of human life and expression than any other. A common thread among all cultures is the reverence they have for the divine nature of this stone, and that is because it stirs a sense of belonging, hope, and peace within the human spirit.

Embodiment and Structure of Jade

Looking over all the different and seemingly disparate uses of jade made researching this stone confusing. The more jade came into my life, the more I wanted. I felt a sincere call to surround myself with this dreamy stone, and I wanted to explore it through all my senses. Most of all, the tactile sensation of jade comforted me on my journey with this gemstone. Jade's final message to us is encoded in this drive to know it through its tangible qualities, which can only be seen when magnified.

Nephrite jade, as described earlier, is comprised of a series of amphibole minerals, primarily tremolite and actinolite. These two minerals form together in tiny strands of crystals that are crumpled and twisted through metamorphic activity. When the jade has finally completed its formation, these fibers are evenly distributed through the entirety of this gemstone, and their interlocking position accounts for jade's incredible toughness. Under great magnification the felted structure of nephrite jade resembles the connective tissues in our own body.[29] Jade works to calm us by acting as a template for our physical body—one infused with peace—so our own tissues will quickly respond to the serene wisdom of jade and return to a state of balance.

If jade is the gate to heaven, peace is the key that unlocks it. A mind overcome by tempestuous emotions and thoughts cannot grant access to the kingdom of the immortals. However, when one's mind and body are completely at ease, then the state of inner peace that results opens the spiritual path beyond measure. In fact, in any spiritual endeavor it can be said that attainment of inner peace should be the goal, and all else is merely a byproduct of peace. For example, working with jade to achieve wealth may indeed increase one's financial abundance; however, seeking peace in the midst of monetary instability can instead yield immeasurable prosperity, both material and immaterial in nature. Choosing to operate from the state of tranquility is one of the single greatest boosts to the ability to manifest your goals. Jade, especially nephrite jade, allows us to deeply root this peace into all levels of our body, just as its own fibrous formation echoes that of our body's tissues. This is what permits jade to effect such deep healing and to attract so many beneficial influences.

Vessels made of jade teach us about embodying the liminal zones in life. Where obsidian helps the seeker find the void and take the first step into it, jade demonstrates that the void is ever-apparent within, and all that is necessary is to embrace the inner void. Peace of mind equates with stillness, such as that which results from surrendering to the moment. This stillness is the cosmic void made manifest, embodied in the core of your being. Where the mirror of obsidian opens your eyes to seeing the void, the jade container trains you to become the empty vessel. Evacuate fear and your ego from your being, and there remains a holiness in the resulting emptiness. In this emptiness one makes room for heaven and the Spirit to enter your being and speak. Only in stillness can you hear the whisperings of heaven.

MEDITATION
ENTERING THE GATEWAY

Jade, like obsidian, is associated with liminal zones. It can facilitate crossing from one plane or level of consciousness into the next. Jade can therefore be used to metaphorically grant access to the heavenly realms. For this exercise, use a piece of jade that is hollow in the center, like a bead, a donut, or a bi. Or you could easily substitute a group of tumbled stones placed in a ring on the table or floor in front of you.

Use the jade as a visual focus. Set your intention for this journey; you can select a specific destination—an outcome or a state of mind—that you would like to realize through the meditation. Once you've set your intention, stare into the empty center of the jade until everything else in the room appears to dissolve. Now imagine this empty center is getting closer and larger, until you can pass right through it. This may take several attempts until you can achieve this. Keep trying until successful.

As you pass through the doorway, imagine that your presence is being purified and uplifted. The jade portal is cleansing, refreshing, and peaceful, like a gentle shower or waterfall. Allow your essence to be awakened and rejuvenated by the virtuous, calming effects of jade. Once on the other side, your consciousness is free to explore. When you have finished, return through the doorway of the jade into normal waking consciousness. Reflect on everything that you have learned, perhaps by journaling your experience.

JADE IN CRYSTAL HEALING

The history of jade's use in healing disease is perhaps one of the oldest of any gemstone. Traditional Chinese medicine cites the stone of heaven as a general tonic and supporter of the kidneys and kidney meridian. The meridians are energy pathways in the body, with specific points that serve as therapy windows for placement of acupuncture needles, acupressure points, and even gemstone placement. The kidney meridian rules the aging process, the eliminatory system, the downward flow of humors of the body, vitality, fertility, and even willpower.[30]

Because of its association with the kidneys, jade can be used to support the various functions of the kidney meridian. On the physical level, jade is first and foremost a stone to bring the entire organism into a state of balance. Its peaceful vibration seeps into the tissues of the body, thereby clearing the way for essence or "essential qi," referred to as *jing* in Chinese medicine, to course through the system. Jade works to help fortify and maintain this vital essence, which in turn leads to longevity and health. We can see the actions of longevity supported through both the structure of jade and its archetypal symbols.

Both varieties of jade, nephrite and jadeite, withstand the test of time far better than most artistic media. These gems are essentially immortal, and their durability and beauty sympathetically confer these same qualities to their wearer. The Chinese as well as other cultures acquainted with jade experienced the stone's connection to eternity and immortality. Wearing jade helps to slow down the aging process and prevents putrefaction after death. This explains why jade has been used as a funerary offering for millennia.

The composition of nephrite in particular can impart an antiaging effect. The structure of this gemstone closely resembles collagen fibers, and for this reason jade can revitalize and rejuvenate the connective tissues.[31] Going back to the seventh century, Chinese nobility fashioned jade into small rollers that could be used on the neck and face for health and beauty. These jade rollers, which provide assistance with lymphatic drainage, decreasing puffiness and reducing fine lines and wrinkles, are making a resurgence in the modern beauty industry. Try massaging the skin of the face in an upward motion with a smooth, polished piece of nephrite if you do not have access to a jade roller.

Jade is considered a natural aid to fertility. This may be in part due to its connection to the kidney meridian, though in reality the symbolism runs much deeper. The many shades of this gemstone are reminiscent of the natural world, and early humankind would have placed special emphasis on those colors they associated with the source of life. For the Olmec and the Maya peoples, blues and greens were especially important. The Olmec treasured blue jade because its color reminded them of maize, while the Maya favored green jades that shone with the same brilliant hue as the sacred wells that supplied water and life to the people. The Maori of New Zealand also connected the color of their native greenstone to the unfurling of new life. Jade, for all people who have known it, has been a symbol of life, vitality, and abundance.

The deep peace that jade emits has therapeutic effects worth noting. Jade is excellent for unwinding the tensions of the body, both because of its structure and the tranquil vibration it brings to its user. Jade instills such a pleasant atmosphere that it can also be used to enhance sleep and provide better rest.

Beyond the physical level, jade is a master healer of the heart center. With jade, the key word is nearly always *peace,* and that holds true for mental and emotional healing, too. From generating a peaceful state of mind jade is then capable of catalyzing forgiveness and compassion. Jade's hardness and fineness belie the perceived softness and remoteness of peace. When used for psychological well-being, this stone enables the peaceful state to become imperturbable. Use it when strength is needed at the heart; jade withstands the passing of eternity, and it therefore helps love last just as long. Symbolically, jade has been given as a gift to bring marital harmony and fidelity. It can be an excellent stone to attract a mate, especially the lavender and pink varieties. Green jade especially brings a sense of joy and lightheartedness to its user.

An Aid to Prosperity Consciousness

One of the premier uses of jade in mental and emotional healing is in the rehabilitation of our relationship with money. As noted, jade is deeply connected to fertility, abundance, and wealth, but all of this is tempered with harmony and serenity. Today, so much of our self-worth is tied to our financial state. In former times, jade, as a royal stone, was often given as tribute to the emperor of China. Qianlong, an emperor who reigned in the eighteenth century, demanded tribute of the finest fei cui, or jadeite of the brightest green, with which he adorned his palace. Jade flowers sprang from jade vases; jade rings were placed on his fingers for archery. Bowls of jade were even used in the preparation of his meals. Due to his obsession with this gemstone, Qianlong earned the moniker "the Jade Emperor."

This imperial gem has very humble beginnings. Formed when mountains are born of colliding tectonic plates, jade is weathered out of mother rock and carried by rivers, where it is broken apart and worn down. This jadeite, when discovered, is often disguised as a plain-looking rock with no apparent value. Larger boulders may be heated over fires until they crack open, thus revealing a gemlike interior. It takes a skilled artisan to reveal the beauty from the drab external appearance of the raw material, and jade only appears to be truly valuable when this beauty is brought to life by polishing. For this reason, jade helps us discover what is truly valuable in life. It reminds us to look deeper than the surface.

Once used as currency, jade now is seen to bestow wealth and good fortune to anyone who possesses a piece. Jade's long association with money and financial success are traditions still upheld by the jade industry today, but the archetypes ask us to look deeper. Jade is not directly responsible for wealth; rather, the stone of heaven brings a divine peace to its wearer. This peace transcends any anxieties or fears about money. Given that jade is used by modern crystal therapists to ameliorate troubles with the emotional center, jade can heal our relationship with money, too.

Jade helps in overcoming the fear of lack, and it instead redirects you to focus on the infinite abundance flowing around you. In most cases, poverty consciousness is a misperception and incorrect valuation of wealth. Jade invites you to ask what truly makes you wealthy. Is it money alone, or is it peace? When inner peace is the goal, abundance follows, and jade prompts this view. Green jade is especially helpful in healing your relationship with money, as it can overcome jealousy, greed, and fear by training the mind to accept peace, compassion, and the abundance of the natural world.

Spiritual Healing Work

Although many are drawn to using nephrite and jadeite for one of the uses already mentioned, the goal of these monoclinic gems is to steer us toward greater spiritual healing. Polishing either variety requires hard work and dedication, and this is not unlike working on your spiritual progress. I have found that jade appears in many spiritual centers in Asia. It is a stone whose peaceful vibration reminds me of the grounds of a holy temple, and this sacred space is where we can cultivate compassion, forgiveness, and nonattachment.

As an ornamental gemstone, jade has been chosen because its toughness allows its beauty to last more or less forever. It is found in association with ancestral artifacts and burial sites, and these occurrences point to a level of healing that can be viewed as generational and karmic. Jade artifacts passed from generation to generation, such as the heitiki of the Maori, allow the healing essence of pounamu, or greenstone, to permeate the entire lineage of its bearer. This begins to resolve the karma carried by the family, thereby freeing the soul and bringing one closer to enlightenment.

Most stones associated with dreaming also bear a connection to karmic healing, and jade is no exception. Jade, as the dream stone, relaxes the mind of its wearer. When taken to bed or used in deep meditation, jade's frequency begins to saturate the aura, from the physical body outward to the higher and more rarified levels of our being. When jade suffuses its energy throughout the causal body, i.e., the karmic body, we can shed and resolve karmic scars that our souls have borne from lifetimes prior to this one. Jade is recommended for past-life recall, and it fosters the emotional detachment necessary to do this kind of healing work without judgment and shame.[32] This makes jade an excellent ally to obsidian when performing any sort of introspective work.

Most important, when I think of jade in the context of spiritual healing I am always reminded of the Buddhist idea of the "fortunate rebirth." This spiritual tradition emphasizes reincarnation and transmigration of the soul. This means that our soul may take on many forms in many lifetimes, from plants and animals to other spiritual beings. Despite the infinite possibilities, it is the human birth that is regarded as the fortunate birth, for only in human incarnation is the soul capable of reaching nirvana, the state of pure bliss and enlightenment. Jade teaches embodiment above all else, and it helps the wearer to become peace itself. Jade truly helps build the bridge from where we are in the material world to where we are headed in the spiritual realms.

Varieties of Jade

Black Jade

Black jade is typically nephrite, and it can be found in various locations, including South America, Australia, and Canada. Most black jade isn't truly black; the color is such an intensely saturated green that it appears to be black until sliced very thin. Black jade is earthy and grounding. It engenders control over the emotions, especially the volatile kind like anger, and it is a deeply nourishing stone for emotional support.[33] It is especially useful for grappling with issues of survival and personal power.[34] When used in dream work, "black jade uses the dream state to process activities and events that are a part of daily living and can give you a great deal of insight into your experience of the mundane world."[35]

Arizona black jade is a recent discovery in the Bradshaw Mountains of the American Southwest. It is primarily composed of nephrite jade and barkevikite, another amphibole mineral. It contains additional iron, mostly as magnetite, which accounts for both the color and the extraordinary density of this jade when compared to other members of the jade family. Arizona black jade is exceptionally grounding and centering; it helps to relieve stress and tension while enhancing focus. It can encourage exploring new directions and avenues in life, allowing the person to feel safe and grounded during the process of discovery. The iron content is especially strengthening, bringing an influence from Mars that leads one to take action and find more passion in life.

Blue Jade

In the truest sense, blue jade isn't actually blue. It occurs as a bluish green or bluish gray coloration, and may be found in both nephrite and jadeite varieties of jade. Blue jade is known for its calming, meditative presence. It is recommended as an aid to meditation as well as for calming fiery energy like "habitual anger, preoccupation with sex, hyperactivity or inflammation."[36] Its combination of earth and air energies makes for an excellent stone to use when objectivity and clear thinking are needed.

Blue nephrite from the Vonsen Ranch, in Marin County, California, is especially useful for chronic pain, clarity in communication, confidence, smooth transitions, and overcoming grief.[37] The Olmec blue variety of jadeite connects one to the Corn Maiden, a goddess of fertility and abundance in traditional Mesoamerica.

Imperial Jade

Imperial jade is a term reserved for only the finest green jadeite. Its color is owed to the presence of chromium as a trace element. The first scientific analysis of jadeite was published in 1863 by mineralogist Augustin Alexis Damour, who had been studying Chinese jades for nearly twenty years.[38] Energetically, jadeite, as imperial jade, is the most refined of all varieties of jade. The source of its pigmentation, chromium, connects it directly to the heart center, and it correspondingly can be used to heal what lies at the heart of most burdens.

Because of its association with the ruling class, the most elite of jades is also the most effective for drawing wealth and manifesting financial abundance. The intensity of its color coupled with the luminous candescence that fine jade exhibits permit this stone to act as a beacon for your goals to manifest. Wear imperial jade to connect to your inner wisdom, especially the wisdom that has accumulated over many lifetimes, in order to exercise good decision-making skills. Imperial jade inspires virtue and tolerance and improves relations among groups of people by building a cohesive identity.[39] In Myanmar (a.k.a. Burma), where most jadeite is found, it was traditionally gathered by jade hunters who searched the riverbeds with their feet to find alluvial deposits of this stone. Jadeite has humble origins, and it keeps our hearts similarly humble even when we find success. This makes it an excellent stone for any leader, executive, or manager.

Japanese Jade

Japanese jade is most often found as jadeite rock rather than pure jadeite. It can appear as mottled veins of green, brown, pink, or other colors in a white rock matrix. It can also appear as fine-grained jadeite of a quality matching that of imperial jade from Myanmar. Like all forms of jade, its energy is very healing and quite dreamlike. This stone reminds me of the ancient Cintamani, the wish-fulfilling gem that appears in different Asian spiritual traditions. One of the three Imperial Regalia of Japan (a.k.a. the Three Sacred Treasures of Japan) is the Yasakani no Magatama; while it has not been seen in public, it is likely that this gemstone is carved from jadeite. The Japanese variants of jade help us find the childlike wonder in our hearts; they impart a lightness and innocence to our dreams and encourage us to make and fulfill our wishes.

Lavender Jade

Lavender and purple jades are among my favorites. These exotic colors can range from dull, dingy shades in either species, to the bright and radiant shades of lavender and lilac best seen in Myanmar jadeite. Of all the colors of jade, these best express the principles of spiritual growth and inner peace. The color of lavender jade is primarily due to trace amounts of manganese, a metal that often produces purple and pink colors in the mineral kingdom. It imparts an air of emotional freedom and trusting one's instincts. This stone is also used to "alleviate emotional hurt and trauma" while teaching "subtlety and restraint in emotional matters."[40]

When found in lavender shades, this stone is perfect for learning to set boundaries because it offers the softness of lavender and the firmness that jade possesses.[41] Lavender combines the colors pink and purple, thereby generating a vibration that is both spiritually expansive and heart-centered. For this reason, lavender jade offers emotional security and inner peace. It combats cynicism, inspires idealism, and displaces skepticism by replacing it with optimism.[42]

Paler shades of lavender jade are associated with the angelic realms, and "instead of being Nature-oriented, however, Lavender Jade's energy is directed toward connection with the cosmic and etheric levels."[43] Darker, purple jade "fills one with mirth and happiness"[44] and can assist in the work of the healer in understanding, transmuting, and releasing the energies of clients without taking on that which is being released or healed.

Lemurian Jade

Lemurian jade is named after the legendary lost continent of Lemuria, said to have once existed in either the Indian Ocean or the Pacific. It is similar in composition to a stone from Guatemala known as galactic gold jade. Lemurian jade is found in two distinct colorations: a dark, blackish background jade that is referred to as "midnight Lemurian jade" and a paler, grayish green gem called "shadow Lemurian jade." Both contain spangles of iron and copper pyrites and quartz among their constituent minerals.

Lemurian jade is found in Peru, from only one source: beneath a functioning copper mine. It is purportedly a combination of two varieties of jade, both nephrite and jadeite. There is no known geological occurrence of the two jade species forming together, and if this claim is true, it is an otherwise impossible phenomenon brought to life by the mysteries of Mother Earth. Lemurian jade is a gem with a genuinely ancient feel to it. The presence surrounding this stone is that of antediluvian dreams and initiation into mysteries unknown today.

Lemurian jade is grounding and expansive. The iron pyrite and chalcopyrite studding the midnight or gray background recall the image of the night sky. While the mineral components of the jade and the pyrite root us firmly in the earth, the visual appearance of the stone encourages the mind and spirit to ascend into the heavens. Lemurian jade teaches you to become the bridge between heaven and earth, and it can initiate you into the Lemurian mysteries. The Lemurian civilization was considered a peaceful, spiritually advanced culture characterized by a profound connection to the natural world and a more intuitive, goddess-oriented set of ideals than the later Atlantean culture. Connecting with this gemstone helps integrate these qualities into your current incarnation. Dreaming with this stone provides a deep connection to the Lemurian culture, and it can also help you recall lifetimes lived on this mysterious lost continent.

Noted crystal healer JaneAnn Dow first introduced this gemstone in 2004; she considered it to be a stone of healing the oversoul. The oversoul here refers to the level of unity wherein all beings' souls connect to one another and to Source. It can resolve karma and act as a catalyst for taking the next step in your spiritual evolution. Try harnessing the energy of this stone during any phase of transition. Midnight Lemurian jade is especially well-suited to working with obsidian, and both midnight and shadow Lemurian jade form the bridge to the archetypes of lapis lazuli, explored in the next chapter. Whether or not these gemstones are comprised of both jade species, they are nevertheless truly one of the most evolved forms of jade available to healers today.

Orange Jade

Orange jade typically is found as either nephrite or jadeite, and its color may be due to the presence of iron and manganese. It carries creativity and vital energy, and channels these energies into the heart. Orange jade is thought to "reduce the tendency to be gullible and naïve," while also energizing the body and offering a protective influence.[45]

Pounamu

New Zealand greenstone is often referred to by its native name, *pounamu*. The Maori people have exclusive rights to this stone, and its collection is therefore restricted. Authentic Maori greenstone carvings are quite expensive. The carvers of New Zealand still employ traditional techniques for polishing this member of the jade family, and they categorize distinct classes of it based on its appearance. Some classes of pounamu are not jade at all and are instead bowenite, a variety of gem-quality serpentine (see page 79). For practical purposes, all types of pounamu, even those that are not nephrite, share the same characteristics due to similar trace elements and a common geologic origin.

Pounamu is the quintessential gemstone of Polynesia. Historically it was reserved for making weapons and ornaments, especially for the ruling class. It is found only in hard-to-reach areas of Aotearoa, the North Island of New Zealand. Each traditional style of carving Maori greenstone indicates one of its spiritual associations. The ceremonial club descended from actual weaponry, the *mere,* is symbolic of the strength and power that greenstone possesses. Like any other type of nephrite, it is tough and difficult to carve and polish due to its density and crystal structure, and so carvings of this jade "indicate the presence of power and personality."[46]

Other traditional carvings include the *koru,* a spiral motif that indicates the cycle of life and new growth; the previously mentioned *hei-tiki,* which conveys an ancestral connection to the guardian archetype; and the *hei-matau,* a stylized fishhook meant to impart strength, safe travel across water, and good luck. Any errant fragment of pounamu could be drilled and strung as an ornament because of the scarcity and sanctity of the material, and it is believed that "contact with pounamu brought benefit to every wearer."[47]

This greenstone is treated with utmost respect, and traditionally the most personal and powerful pieces used in healing were usually those given as gifts rather than purchased. Among the Maori, the assistance of a shaman was used to locate the right stone for the wearer. It is a symbol of peace, healing, and good fortune, revered and respected by the native people of New Zealand because it "holds the memories of the past and knowledge of the future. It receives messages and passes them on to its keeper."[48]

Red Jade

Red jade is a potent stone for healing and detoxifying the physical body. It expands the emphasis of jade's energy from the kidney meridian to include the circulatory system as well. The red color is nearly always due to iron compounds, and iron is associated with the planet Mars in astrology. This active, courageous force drives the healing presence of jade to flow throughout the system on all levels. Red jade can be used to overcome addictions, as well as to impart physical strength to the body.[49] It does so by inviting the Martian influences into the body's tissues, including connective tissues and muscles, through jade's sympathetic resonance with these parts of the body.

White Jade

Compared to all its cousins, white jade is perhaps the most archetypal of the virtues—such as those extolled by Confucius, including kindness, truthfulness, humility, intelligence, and justice—and of peace. White jade is a result of a lack of trace elements that are otherwise responsible for the many colors in which both nephrite and jadeite are encountered. Because of this, white jade is akin to a blank canvas. It stills the mind, and to me represents the Zen principle of "beginner's mind." White stones are typically associated with spiritual pursuits, and this gemstone is no exception. "White jade is a highly spiritual vibration that can be used to stimulate the precognitive faculty which is sometimes very active in the dream state or to enhance a talent for lucid dreaming."[50]

White jade can also filter distractions while "emphasizing the best possible result."[51] This snow white rock helps one find the intersection of spirituality and practicality. Meditating with white jade and wearing it in daily life helps the spiritual aspirant seek opportunity and grace every day. Although it is highly spiritual in nature, this member of the jade family can also make it "easy to see objective reality," which makes it an especially good stone for daydreamers.[52] Although it lacks the trace elements that ground its energy like other jades, this stone is still exceptionally peaceful, and it is capable of helping you have better awareness and attention in the present moment.

Yellow Jade

Most yellow jade being marketed today is actually yellow serpentine. Nevertheless, true yellow nephrite and jadeite are available. I have found yellow jade to be very cheerful in its disposition, and it is likely to impart this sense of happy contentedness to its wearer. Though mellower than orange or red jade, yellow jade is still energizing, and it resonates with the sacral and solar plexus chakras. Its connection to the sacral chakra makes it especially good for exploring relationships with those around us; it "teaches the interconnectedness of all life" while simultaneously giving a "sense of understanding relating to the opposite sex."[53] It can similarly be used for promoting empathy and understanding of anyone, regardless of gender.

All varieties of jade work to heal the kidney function, but yellow jade is the most effective for healing or supporting any aspect of the eliminatory system, including the kidneys, bladder, skin, and lungs. Each of these organs eliminates metabolic wastes from the body, and yellow jade can assist their function by releasing any tension or apprehension, both physically and psychologically.

Related Stones

Many other gem materials are marketed as jade, although they are neither jadeite nor nephrite. Generally speaking, most of these minerals convey healing qualities similar to those of jade, and some are related to jade either in composition or in formation.

Actinolite

Actinolite is one of the two constituent minerals of nephrite jade. Additionally, it can be found as dense aggregates of fibrous, prismatic crystals and as inclusions of similar crystals in quartz and other minerals. Using actinolite provides an expansion of the energy bodies and a connection to All That Is.[54] It is also protective; the fibrous structure of actinolite disperses unwanted energy. This mineral formation can also "seal the edges" of the energy bodies, or biomagnetic sheath,[55] and the fibrous and columnar form of the crystals is excellent for amplifying the communication between all of the bodies, physical and energetic; the crystals act like wires to provide clear, uninterrupted exchange, thereby encouraging all parts of our being to work in harmony for total wellness and health.

Actinolite is sometimes found in quartz. When this occurs, the fibers themselves tend to be a greenish color, sometimes with a metallic sheen. They encourage a connection to the natural world and can help you listen to and interpret the messages of nature. It is also "helpful when you have lost your way and are looking for new direction."[56] When densely packed and arranged in a parallel fashion, actinolite may create a cat's-eye effect in quartz; these gemstones are highly protective and visionary. Use them to unlock creativity and to overcome any sort of obstacle on your path.

Aventurine

Aventurine is a massive formation of quartz that is composed of fine grains of clear-to-cloudy quartz and inclusions of other minerals that provide it with its color and a degree of sparkle. Aventurine may be found in many colors, with green being the most common. Green aventurine may superficially resemble jade, but it is a different stone altogether. Aventurine has long been considered a lucky stone, often recommended for gambling and winning money. It represents nurturing the self and growing new projects, and it is frequently used to assist physical healing by uplifting and detoxifying the physical body. Energetically, aventurine shares several similarities with jade. Both confer good fortune and can be used to facilitate financial gain and true abundance. The fine-grained composition of aventurine is similar to that of jadeite, and both can be considered stabilizing, nurturing stones.

Chrome Diopside

Diopside is a pyroxene mineral that is closely related to jadeite. In fact, jadeite from many locations may contain a large amount of diospide in its composition. Diopside may be green to brown, as well as black. Some massive varieties exhibit asterism when polished. While all forms of diopside have their own personality, only those containing chromium will be discussed here, for they share this element and its spiritual influences with imperial jadeite.

Chrome diopside has a rich, emerald green color and a brilliant refractive index. When visibly free of inclusions it makes a delightful faceted stone. Chrome diopside lights a spiritual flame within its wearer. The vibrant green light of this stone initiates artistic expression, and it can allow for a profound appreciation of nature. Chrome diopside is an excellent stone for overcoming writer's block, and it can yield inspiration in analytical pursuits, such as problem-solving.

Maw Sit Sit

This rare gemstone, also known as jade-albite, hails from Myanmar, and is a close cousin to jadeite, which is found nearby. Maw sit sit is named after the location where it was first found, in the foothills of the Himalayas. It is a metamorphic rock composed of pyroxenes, including jadeite, diopside, and kosmochlor, with albite feldspar and chromite among the other minerals present. The mineral in greatest abundance is kosmochlor, a silicate of sodium and chromium. The composition of maw sit sit was decoded in 1963 by Swiss gemologist Eduard Gubelin.

An attractive and rare gemstone, very little literature exists on the healing properties of maw sit sit. It shares many compositional features with jade, and it forms under similar metamorphic circumstances. Because of this, the properties of jade apply to this Myanmar rock. Additionally, this gemstone "gives us a special gift. We feel hope that we will find accomplishment."[57] Its complex structure is even more difficult to picture than that of either member of the jade family, therefore, maw sit sit has mastery over complexity. It can shed light and understanding on where we fit into the bigger picture. The result of this, much like working with jade, is profound peace. Maw sit sit can help you find joy in all your endeavors, while it is truly an ally for spiritual and emotional healing. Its chief component mineral, kosmochlor, was actually first identified in a meteorite, giving it a name derived from the German word *kosmisch,* meaning "cosmic." The energy of maw sit sit is otherworldly, and it can comfort those who feel out of place on planet Earth.

Prehnite

Prehnite is an uncommon mineral that is occasionally mistaken for jade. Most prehnite is a green color, and it is commonly found as botryoidal, or grapelike, forms. Some examples, especially those from Australia, seem to have a candescent quality, and they are occasionally termed "sun jade" by dealers. Many specimens are peppered with blades of green epidote crystals within. Polished, most prehnite will be a yellowish green, and its luster should be pearly.

Prehnite has been recommended by modern crystal therapists for dream work. While no ancient literature on this stone exists, it has been said to enhance the recall of one's dreams, which is not unlike the properties of jade. This unusual green gemstone is also considered to be the stone of healing the healer, and it is associated with the archetype of the wounded healer, Chiron, from Greek mythology. More recently, prehnite has been suggested as being the symbiotic partner of nephrite jade. The energy of prehnite is softening, and it allows the physical body to become more receptive and flexible to positive change. Because of this, jade is more able to perform its function; prehnite can be said to open the doorway to benefitting from jade by making the energy patterns of the body more permeable.[58] Using the two in tandem is especially suited to any work centered on repairing physical tissue, or for integrating jade's peaceful energy into our entire system. If you feel stuck with jade, as if you've reached a plateau with no further progress, partnering it with prehnite can accelerate and deepen its benefits, thus enabling your work to proceed.

Serpentine

No discussion of jade is complete without addressing its most frequent competitor and mimic, serpentine. When serpentine is marketed as jade, it is commonly referred to as "new jade," although it is also sometimes called "false jade," "Soochow jade," "Mexican jade," and "Shanghai jade." Serpentine actually refers to a group of minerals rather than a single mineral type. Each member of the serpentine group is a hydrous magnesium iron phyllosilicate. They vary in composition, with chromium, manganese, cobalt, and nickel being frequent substitutions in their structures. Serpentine minerals form in metamorphic serpentinite rocks, and they are soft enough to carve, with a rich history as ornamental stones.

Most varieties of serpentine are green to brown in color, with different degrees of translucency and opacity. Most varieties marketed as new jade are fairly translucent to subtransparent. Other varieties may be altogether opaque. As described earlier, serpentine almost always occurs in association with jadeite, and they are excellent stones to use in tandem. Serpentine is softer and lighter than either nephrite or jadeite, and no member of the serpentine group ever forms as single crystals. The inherent softness and lightness of serpentine makes it a gentler healing stone than jade, especially when working with the archetypes associated with self-reflection and refinement.

Overall, serpentine is an excellent stone for physical healing, as it imparts strength and action to the immune system. Named for its resemblance to snakeskin, serpentine is symbolically linked to the rising of the kundalini, the serpentlike energy that resides in the base of the spine and moves upward when awakened. Serpentine is a very ancient-feeling stone with close connections to nature. Many types of serpentine also contain inclusions of magnetite and other magnetic ores. Because of this, it "acts as a recorder of Earth shifts as told through the geological and energetic patterns of this metamorphic stone."[59] Connecting with this stone provides deep connection to the earth, and for this reason it is "a powerful stone for Earth Healers and Mages who focus their energies on understanding and assisting the planet through its current transformations."[60] Jadeite takes advantage of the low density of serpentine in order to rise from the mantle to the surface of the earth; it is essentially a hitchhiker on serpentine's journey. Allow this metamorphic stone to carry you to the next stop on your journey as you, too, begin your skyward ascent.

Transvaal Jade

Transvaal jade, sometimes called "African jade," is the name for massive formations of hydrogrossular garnet. This member of the garnet family may also contain up to 25 percent of another mineral, zoisite, accounting for the hydroxide ions that substitute for some of the silica in its composition. Found only in microcrystalline masses, Transvaal jade is named after its place of origin, Transvaal, in the Republic of South Africa. Typically, it is found in colors such as white, green, orange, and pink, and a single vein may possess a combination of these and other colors.

Transvaal jade crystallizes in the cubic crystal system. As such, it is an excellent stone for building foundations and encouraging organization. Garnets are gemstones typically associated with grounding, prosperity, and physical health, and these qualities are present in this jade simulant from Africa. It is also excellent for birthing insight in the face of adversity and is recommended for the "treatment of disorders of the veins, restrictions in energy flow, problems of the heart (both physical and emotional) . . . dysfunction due to trauma, and irregularities in the area of the throat."[61]

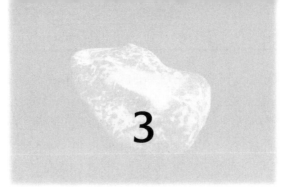

3

LAPIS LAZULI

The Starry Sky and the All-Seeing Eye

Imagine a deep indigo–colored sky, with wispy swirls of clouds and mist; glittering starlight has begun to filter into view. Now imagine this scene unfolding before your eyes as you break through hard stone to reveal an ultramarine gemstone that has captivated humanity since its discovery. The earth has many treasures, and few have had the cultural impact of lapis lazuli, a gemstone whose very name is a nod to its heavenly disposition and spiritual value.

The history of lapis lazuli stretches back into prehistory, with its use as a gem material spanning nine thousand years. Cultures all around the globe have all been beguiled by its color and suitability as a carving medium—Mesopotamia and Egypt, the Far East, North Africa, Europe, and even in the Andes Mountains of South America. Its name is derived from the Latin word for stone, *lapis,* and the Persian word for blue, *lajuvard* or *lazhuvard,* which can be traced to Arabic, then to Latin.[1] The Arabic *lazaward* refers not only to the color blue; it also means "sky" and "heaven," creating a solid link to the abode of the gods at the very mention of this gem's name. In most cultures acquainted with this celestial stone it has been similarly connected to the deep azure sky with stars dotted and clouds streaked across it.

Lapis lazuli is a metamorphic rock rather than being a single mineral or gemstone. It is comprised of three primary minerals, with a wide range of accessory minerals that may be included in its composition. Primarily comprised of lazurite, lapis consists of lesser amounts of golden pyrite and white calcite. The brilliant blue of this stone is owed to its sulfur and sodium content, while varying amounts of complementary and contrasting colors are due to any number of impurities. Other colors that may be found in the matrix of lapis lazuli include indigo, violet, green, red, white, brown, and black, in addition to the typical white and gold amid the blue.

Lazurite is a member of the sodalite group of minerals. It has recently been reclassified as a variety of the mineral hauyne, having lost its classification as a separate mineral species. Lazurite is a cubic mineral and is generally opaque. It forms in metamorphic environments as limestone is gradually transformed into new minerals. It occurs in very few locations in the world, with even fewer producing good-quality lapis lazuli. Lazurite often occurs in association with other members of the sodalite group, including nosean, hauyne, and sodalite itself. Their compositions are all similar, and they share a cubic geometry.

Calcite, a calcium carbonate mineral, is found in differing amounts in lapis, with the finest gemstones displaying little to no calcite whatsoever. It is present as whitish streaks when visible and is generally present at the microscopic level even when it cannot be seen. "Under a microscope thin sections show a matrix of calcite enclosing numerous blue and colorless grains."[2] Pyrite, an iron sulfide commonly called "fool's gold," provides metallic dots and bands of golden yellow, which contrasts with the deep blue of lazurite and resembles stars in the sky. The accessory minerals in lapis lazuli typically consist of any combination of diopside, amphibole, feldspar, mica, and other silicates.[3] They are responsible for the mottled effect of the blues and other colors present in a given sample of lapis. The variation in colors and patterns can even indicate a specimen's origin, although such identification will require a well-trained eye.

Lapis forms under unique conditions of metamorphic activity. It began its journey at the bottom of the oceans. Organic material such as the skeletons and shells of aquatic organisms that lived millions of years ago eventually formed a limestone bedrock from the action of sedimentation and compression. This host rock was eventually subjected to the processes that form mountains, and through these cataclysmic forces the chemical elements found in the limestone shifted, swirled, and reorganized themselves into new mineral structures. Eventually, lapis lazuli rose from the depths of the sea and was reborn at the heart of the highest mountain ranges such as the Himalayas, one of the most important sources; in this way dull rock gave way to a heavenly gem.

This metamorphic activity causes lapis lazuli to exhibit foliation, a more or less banded appearance found in many samples of this stone. Foliation occurs as minerals in the parent rock are exposed to greater and greater amounts of heat and pressure. The different minerals dissolve and are compressed into discrete bands during the rock-forming processes. As the processes continue, these bands can be further subjected to orogeny, the process of birthing mountains, among other types of metamorphoses, and these can intermingle the once-banded minerals into the more recognizable swirls in some specimens of lapis lazuli.

Lapis lazuli, or more specifically lazurite, can be found in the highest mountains of only nine countries in the world. They are: Afghanistan, Canada, Chile, India, Italy, Myanmar, Russia, Pakistan, and the United States. Because boundaries have been redrawn throughout history, lapis has been ascribed to other countries in the Middle East that now lie within the borders of Afghanistan.

LAPIS LAZULI FROM
THE ANCIENT WORLD TO TODAY

Like jade, lapis lazuli is frequently described as a gemstone of heaven. It was famed throughout antiquity for its noble color with celestial connotations. Beads are thought to be the earliest ornamental use of this gemstone, and they can be found among the grave goods of many cultures in and around the cradle of civilization—Mesopotamia, Sumer, Egypt, and Persia. These and other great cultures admired lapis and valued it above all other gems. It was prized for its soothing qualities, for healing afflictions of the eye, and for providing protection. It was considered to be "insurance for the afterlife" because it was thought to ensure a safe voyage post mortem to the realms of paradise.[4]

In Europe, during the Middle Ages and the Renaissance, the fame of lapis grew not only from its curative powers and beauty as an ornamental stone but also because it was a prized source of the costliest of blue pigments, ultramarine, which was reserved for illuminated manuscripts and for the robes of the holiest of figures on canvas and fresco alike. Michelangelo used this legendary blue in the Sistine Chapel. The rarest of blue pigments could only be made at extreme cost, and lapis was therefore used sparingly, for sacred art, and only rarely for secular art.

The identity of this stone has been confused over millennia, for it is the stone known in biblical times as sapphire, or *sappir* in Hebrew texts. Later called *sapphirus,* this sacred blue stone formed part of the foundation of the ancient Hebrews' Second Temple, as well as adorned the high priest's breastplate, and it may have been among the precious stones on the Ark of the Covenant. Because this heavenly gem material was traded extensively throughout the Middle East and the surrounding regions, it is no surprise that ancient religious texts from the Hebrew Bible to the Epic of Gilgamesh allude to it; indeed, this holy stone and its virtues were praised by all the cultures that knew it.

On the other side of the world, the lapis found in the Andean Mountains was known to native peoples, including the Diaguitas, Molle, Chimu, and the Incas. Pre-Columbian cultures prized this blue rock and harnessed its beauty for use in beads, masks, and carvings of the condor. It was found in a limestone matrix high in the mountains and is still mined there today. Chilean lapis is sometimes referred to as "denim lapis" because its colors and textures resemble that of an acid-washed pair of blue jeans; the difference between the South American and Afghani lapis is the result of a higher calcite content.

The tradition of venerating lapis continued through history. Catherine the Great is known to have commissioned a room paneled in fine Russian lapis lazuli because of her great love of the stone. Carl Fabergé, of the famous House of Fabergé, made use of lapis in creating the famed Fabergé "Imperial" Easter eggs, gifts from Czar Alexander III to his wife. The tradition was continued by Czar Nicholas's successor, and the prized stone of heaven ornamented numerous royal eggs.[5]

The Crystal Craze of the Twentieth Century

No text on the spiritual value of gemstones from the early part of the twentieth century omits this precious blue stone. Because ancient peoples placed such great value on lapis lazuli, when the crystal healers of the 1970s and '80s began to work with it, they too, considered it a precious stone with distinctive qualities. The earlier works from this time period mostly quote from classical sources, although they add the modern twist of chakra associations to the many uses of lapis.

Among crystal healers and gemstone enthusiasts at the onset of the crystal craze, lapis garnered more and more attention due to the importance of it among Edgar Cayce's readings. Books detailing the power of stones as taught by the Sleeping Prophet give special regard to lapis lazuli. He recommended the stone for psychic development, safety amid dangerous circumstances, and spiritual development.[6]

Most authors regard this stone as especially beneficial for the throat and third-eye chakras, and several caution users as to its potency. In time, lapis would be recognized as one of the few gemstones to manifest the indigo ray. In gemstone therapy, the seven colors are considered to manifest as archetypal rays of energy, each one carried by one or more specific gems (see box). Of the seven color rays, indigo is believed to be the most deficient on our planet, and so it is crucial to the spiritual evolution of Earth. Although not the main carrier for this indigo ray, lapis lazuli provides much-needed supporting indigo energy.

Lapis lazuli has remained a trusted and prized stone among crystal healers. Lapis is known to vary in color dramatically based on quality and source, but it consistently comes to us bearing a deep indigo color. Because of the relative scarcity of indigo stones and the indigo ray on our planet, lapis can be an excellent aid to anchoring the indigo ray and all that it represents as we navigate through these changing times.

Introducing the Rays

The seven rays are an occult philosophy originating centuries ago, with several permutations in use today. In brief, the rays are seven archetypal forces, considered to be individuated aspects of God or Source. Each of the rays is typically assigned one or more colors, a planetary ruler, gemstones, and other symbols. Each ray typically extends its influence through dynamic functions associated with that ray, thus corresponding to different aspects and activities in life. Some of the most popular systems of the seven rays include those of Alice Bailey and Mark and Elizabeth Clare Prophet.

There is no definitive list of colors, planets, effects, or gems that spans all the systems of the rays. Throughout the text you will see references to the rays as they are described by different schools of thought with regard to the seven archetypal stones. Studying the rays in depth is beyond the scope of this book, as there are centuries of teachings and commentary on the rays, many of which contradict one another. Thus the information on the rays in this text has been limited to discussions relevant to the various stones' archetypes.

Of special note is a system known as the color rays, which was introduced in the 1980s as gemstone therapy was developed. Several chapters in this text relate various gemstones to the rays of gem therapy. The rays of gem therapy are considered to be refractions of the White Light of God, not unlike other philosophies. Each color ray traditionally has a single gemstone carrier, which acts as an anchor for the ray on our planet, although some rays have additional stones to support their missions. Because this system is an easily comprehensible, stand-alone system, each of the rays will be outlined in brief.*

The red ray is carried by ruby, and it represents deriving strength through the emotions. It supplies motion and nourishes the aspects of the physical body responsible for gross movement and physical power, such as the muscles, tendons, fascia, and especially cardiac tissue.

The orange ray, carried by carnelian, exudes vital energy and optimism. It is connected to cycles of cause and effect, and conveys a balancing force in healing. It is also strongly connected to cycles and timing. In the physical body the orange ray fuels metabolic activities, the immune system, endocrine system, and adipose tissue.

The yellow ray is officially carried by yellow sapphire, although citrine acts as a secondary stone for working with its energy. The yellow ray supports elimination and finds strength in spiritual potential. In the body this ray rules the eliminatory organs, including the digestive system, kidneys, skin, and some functions of the lungs and liver.

The green ray expresses itself through understanding the material world as resulting directly from the spiritual world. Carried by emerald, the green ray paves the way to total physical mastery and health as a result of this spiritual orientation. It rules the visceral organs and any reparative processes in the body, as well as supporting the health of the brain.

The blue ray is carried by blue sapphire, and its influence lies in the realm of the mind. The blue ray nourishes mental processes and leads to inner-world mastery and communication. In the physi-

---

*More information on the color rays can be found in Michael Katz's books *Wisdom of the Gemstone Guardians* (141–43) and *Gemstone Energy Medicine* (40–42).

cal body it strengthens channels of communication and flow, such as blood vessels, the myelin sheaths around nerve cells, the brain, and the sensory organs.

The indigo ray is carried by transparent, crystalline forms of sodalite, although non-gem-quality sodalite and lapis support its mission. This is the ray of intuition, as it grants access to understanding the inner form or pattern in a situation. Because of its insight into the structure of a situation, it also rules structural elements in the physical body, such as bones, cartilage, and ligaments.

Finally, the violet ray (often called the purple ray in gemstone therapy) has historically been carried by amethyst. Because of shifts in planetary consciousness, a new gemstone carrier has made itself known: purple tourmaline. The final ray oversees currents of wisdom. Its influence brings spiritual harmony and seeks out limitations so that one can overcome obstacles through spiritual wisdom. In the physical body the violet ray is also responsible for the health of the nervous system.

Gemstone therapy recognizes two more rays, the pink ray, which nourishes the health of the emotional body, and the white ray, which is expressed when all the seven main rays shine in perfect balance. The pink ray is carried by pink tourmaline, and the white ray can be expressed through colorless beryl, clear quartz, and certain high-quality diamonds. An in-depth examination of the color rays of gemstone therapy yields many similarities to other systems of rays, and it can be considered complementary to working with virtually any system of healing.

LAPIS LAZULI AS AN ARCHETYPE: THE STARRY SKY

Lapis brings its owner in touch with the expanse of the celestial sphere because of its uncanny resemblance to a star-studded sky. To gaze at a piece of fine lapis is like staring into the firmament. Throughout human history lapis has been held in high regard because of this likeness to the heavenly realms, and for this reason in order to satisfy the high demand for the heavenly stone it was carried great distances regardless of the inherent perils of early trade routes. The cool, bright blue of lazurite is highlighted by the shimmering gold of pyrite "stars." Calcite "clouds" and "nebulae" add nuance to each and every piece.

The exceptionally vivid color of lapis lazuli stood out among the other gemstones accessible to the populations of the ancient world, and for this reason it gained deeply spiritual connotations and came to be associated with the divine. Deities of many cultures are viewed as residing in heaven, and lapis evokes the image of the residence of the gods and goddesses. For this reason, this sacred blue rock has been frequently unearthed in early burials among funerary offerings, much like jade. Earliest finds of lapis are generally beads, and they are believed to have a protective function for the living as well as the dead.

Not long after the initial fascination with lapis began it became de rigueur on all holy images. Ancient statues can be found with lapis ornaments, from eyes and beards to thrones and crowns. Ancient goddesses such as Inanna, Isis, Ishtar, and Astarte, often considered to be aspects of the primal Mother Goddess, are all known for having lapis among the goods offered to them and adorning their iconic figures. Additionally, deities of the celestial realms such as Sin, the lunar bull god of Babylonia and Sumer, were frequently connected with lapis lazuli. Several deities of ancient Egypt were intimately linked to lapis lazuli. Nuit, the goddess of the night sky, was depicted as deep blue and covered in stars to resemble this holy stone, while the eyes of Horus and Ra were crafted from the stone of heaven. Even Thoth, a lunar deity and scribe, was sometimes connected to lapis lazuli. Solar gods of Egypt all seemed to have associations with this stone too because of the connection to the cosmic scarab, which will be explored in detail later.

As the stone made its way to the Mediterranean and the Far East, pigments of lapis lazuli adorned temples in Knossos, and lapis was used to venerate the Temple of Heaven in China.[7] Ultramarine pigments were similarly reserved for sacred use. Depictions of the Buddha and various bodhisattvas in Asia, as well as the robes of the Madonna and Christ Child, were resplendent with deep blue lapis hues. Haloes of saints and angels radiated an unearthly celestial light from the very same source.

Lapis was powerfully protective to ancient peoples around the world. Its heavenly energy represented purity, peace, and all that is holy. The innate holiness of lapis repels the unholy, much like the way vampires flee from crosses. In light of this, anyone lucky or wealthy enough to own lapis was believed to be safe from harm of all sorts, although lapis's effects are much more than simply deflective. The celestial energy to which it is linked by sympathetic resonance is of a much greater amplitude than negative influences. When two vibrating fields come together, despite the varying frequency of each field, that which has the greater amplitude always wins, bringing the other into harmony with it. In other words, lapis does not merely shield its owner from negative energy; it brings fields of harmful energy into sympathy with the heavenly, thus transforming them into positive influences. This paves the way for transcending the illusion of separation, in which each of us appears to be a separate, discrete, individualized entity. Lapis does not erect a barrier to keep others out, but instead it embraces the divine potential of all energy fields and therefore all sentient beings.

Returning to the Stars

Lapis opens the heart and mind to the infinite possibility and endless expanse of the starry sky. While it is an earthy stone as judged by its composition and dense, opaque appearance, lapis frees the spirit and engenders hope. It teaches one to soar to new heights, as if one's soul had wings with which it could traverse the night sky. Ancient people made this association with lapis from its earliest uses, and today it is possible to learn the same freedom through the lapis lazuli.

Since the earliest days of humankind there is has been a primal longing to seek out starlight and take flight. Ancient legends are rife with tales of flying machines, birdlike deities, and origin myths that trace our lineage back to the stars. Lapis serves as a pathway back to the stars, and it reminds all who gaze at its bespangled beauty that all life is descended from the stars. For many people, especially now, life on planet Earth causes extreme anxiety, and countless people walking the spiritual path often feel displaced as they must embrace an earthly existence and an earthly body. Dreams of flying, experiences of extraterrestrial contact, and a longing for a return to an off-world "homeland" can be symptomatic of a need for more stellar energy in one's life.

Ultimately, lapis is a reminder that despite our earthly bodies we have cosmic origins. Our bodies and our planet are ultimately made from the same matter that once belonged to stars; therefore, it is our natural inclination to want to return to the primal state of starlight. Humankind, as descendants of Creator, are born of the celestial sphere, and as we reacquaint ourselves with our divine origins, a persistent yearning to reintegrate with the light from which we come takes root within. Lapis treats this sensation of separation and a longing for completeness by reminding us of the hope that dwells within our hearts. It grants insight into the path to which we aspire.

Divine Connections

Throughout world history, lapis lazuli has been reserved for the veneration of deities. The ancient gods and goddesses of the stone of heaven tend to be the sky gods, star goddesses, and keepers of paradise and the celestial bodies. Nuit, the star goddess of Egypt, and Sin, the moon bull of the cradle of civilization, are both associated with lapis. In the Far East, the Temple of Heaven, in present-day Beijing, was considered the domain of the immortals. Even the paradise of Mahayana Buddhism was fabled to have sands of lapis lazuli, which feature in the sand mandalas made by Tibetan monks.

The archetype of the starry sky is the domain of the Cosmic Mother. The womb of the Great Mother is as vast as the night sky, and within it was conceived the entirety of the cosmos. To the Egyptians, she was known under the guise of Isis, Nuit, and Ma'at. In Assyria and Babylonia, this primal Mother was Ishtar, and her Babylonian counterpart was Inanna. To the ancient Canaanites she was Astarte. For all she was the goddess of love, sex, magic, and motherhood. This widespread worship of the Cosmic Mother represents the fascination with the birth of humankind. Long before science began to explore the origins of life, mythology introduced ancient humans to their maker. The goddesses of the mystery traditions are the archetypal mothers of the universe; they begat the stars, moons, and suns, as well as our planet and all life on it. This parallels our own celestial lineage, for in countless traditions humankind is viewed as being the progeny of Creator—even so far as to be made in "his" image in the patriarchal Abrahamic faiths.

In the ancient mystery traditions, the womb of the goddess is a celestial cauldron out of which all things are birthed. Obsidian may be the primal void, the prima materia not yet differentiated. Lapis lazuli represents the Great Mother who gives it form, as well as the midwife who ushers the explicate order into creation. Even modern science suggests that we come from the cosmic cauldron, as the birth of the universe began with the Big Bang; it is said that all matter we see in our galaxy is a result of the massive explosion of a dying star. It gave birth to our sun, the planets, and even life on Earth. Lapis, a stone found deep in the heart of the highest mountains, reminds us that even the humblest of rocks owes its lineage to the stars.

One particular divine mother whose cult was known throughout the ancient world was Isis. She and her son, Horus, were worshipped by people throughout Egypt's history, and they were eventually adopted by the Hellenistic world. Figurines of carved lapis lazuli depict the two seated on a throne, while later iconography represented the *udjat,* or Eye of Horus, carved from the most holy of blue stones. One of Isis's many titles was "the throne of Horus," for as an infant he is often shown seated on her lap. Horus was a sky god, traditionally represented by the head of a hawk. The earliest of cult symbols from religious movements in predynastic Egypt are hawks, some of which were carved from lapis lazuli.[8] The sky was the domain of birds and gods alike, for it was the unknown height and mystery that early religions sought to cross through initiation into secret orders.

Another mother of divine importance is Mary, mother of Jesus of Nazareth. The Madonna, as she is known, was often painted in robes of holy blue, with the infant Jesus enthroned on her lap just as Horus sat on the lap of Isis. The ancient sapphirus, which we know to be lapis lazuli, was a stone regarded as sacred to the Madonna. "Konrad von Hamburg made the sapphire the symbol of hope exemplified by the Virgin Mary in his poem Anulus, written circa 1350."[9] Even today, Mary is sometimes connected to the role of mother of the stars in her role as Mary, Queen of the Universe.

The archetype of the starry sky yields its domain not only to the Cosmic Mother. Many sky gods, who are often solar gods, also claim the sphere of the heavens as their own. Solar deities are starlike in their own right, for the sun is but a star close enough to give us daylight.

MEDITATION

REMEMBERING YOUR CELESTIAL ORIGINS

Choose a piece of lapis that you can hold or wear for this meditation. A strand of beads or a pendant that falls on or near your heart is ideal. Settle into a comfortable, quiet space with your stone and prepare to meditate. While holding or wearing your lapis lazuli, imagine that you are staring up at the night sky. Allow the stone to lift you heavenward, so that you travel among the stars.

You are met by radiant beings of light, clothed in robes of ultramarine. These are your personal guides and guardians, and they want to help you remember your celestial heritage. They may share wisdom, offer a gift, or simply stay with you in comfortable silence. Keep an open heart as you stay with these beings of light; they remind you that you are just as luminous as they are. As you breathe in harmony with them, your lungs are filled with the starlight they emanate. Breathe that light into every cell, every molecule, every particle of your being. The light nourishes you and awakens your cellular memory of your noble, divine origins.

Thank the beings once you have finished and gently permit your awareness to return to the earthly plane. Hold your lapis to your heart center and sit in grateful silence as you integrate the messages or energies you received on the spiritual plane. Once you feel grounded and centered, breathe deeply and return your awareness to the room around you.

The Scarab and the Path of the Sun

The starlight and associated hope that are literally written in stone by way of lapis lazuli connect us to the Heavenly Father as much as to the Cosmic Mother. Solar deities were the focus of much of ancient Egyptian myth and magic. Horus, Ra, and Kephera all stand as gods of the sun, and each has been worshiped with offerings of lapis lazuli. Early monotheistic cults, which may have given rise to the subsequent patriarchal Abrahamic traditions, center around the worship of the sun. In Christianity and Judaism, the central deity is a father figure who is analogous to the Source.

The scarab is an iconic image that is featured in Egyptian symbolism throughout the dynasties. Scarabs are beetles, specifically dung beetles. The lowly scarab rolls animal feces in spherical shapes into which it lays its eggs. The beetles can be seen herding these balls across the desert sands, tracing the same east-to-west pathway that the sun also follows. To the inhabitants of the desert, the sun was often imagined as a gleaming sphere being rolled across the starry sky by a giant scarab. The sun is the source of light, heat, and energy, and as such it is ultimately the great life-giver of our planet; because of this, those initiated into the mysteries recognized the great power inherent in scarabaeiform amulets.

The scarab played a role in many aspects of Egyptian life; it was at once holy and protective. The most sacred medium out of which it could be carved was lapis lazuli. Of the many types of scarabs carved by ancient artisans, the heart scarab was the pinnacle of them all. It was placed among the wrappings of the embalmed body and served to protect the heart of the deceased. To the ancient Egyptians, the heart was the most important of all the organs, the only one placed back inside the body after embalming a deceased person. The heart was considered the "seat of thought,"[10] and for this reason lapis was chosen as the finest material for heart scarabs. It exerts a celestial influence over the heart while also engendering peace and hope. Evidence of analogous charms carved in the form of human hearts exist even in later dynasties.[11]

The daily path of the sun was a source of hope and renewal within ancient mystery-school teachings. The scarab's use of the dung ball as a form of the cosmic womb out of which its larvae are born hearkens to the womb of the Mother Goddess. The sun travels across the sky and dies each day at dusk, only to be born again the following morning. Similarly, the scarab became a symbol of regeneration and resurrection; this makes it the perfect accompaniment into the afterlife.

The heart is central for admittance into heaven in Egyptian mythology. The Egyptian Book of the Dead contains a number of spells to ensure the safe passage into the afterlife, one of which is a spell using lapis lazuli to ensure that one's heart not work against its owner.[12] The dead harness the power of lapis to renew the heart and resurrect the spirit among the stars.

Unifying the Heart and the Mind

Today, one of the main purposes for using lapis lazuli in a healing setting is for harmonizing the heart and the mind.[13] While most people associate lapis with the third-eye chakra and the mental-spiritual realms, it gains access to these higher realms by entering our emotional bodies via the heart center. As the true seat of thought, the heart is our most important center for spiritual evolution.

Lapis lazuli opens the heart to the "height of celestial hope"[14] and assists in the release of negative memories and karma accrued from past lives. It works to bring the mind and the emotions into greater cooperation, thereby fostering a new consciousness within the spiritual seeker. This becomes the seed for Christ Consciousness, which will be discussed in greater detail later in this book. With this new, elevated state of consciousness comes renewed vision. Nestled among the stars, one's perspective widens to encompass a greater view. This in turn accounts for the increased psychic awareness and intuitive abilities so often credited to lapis.

Resurrection

Beyond the jade gateway, the realm of lapis lazuli guides the spiritual aspirant to new heights. Lapis serves as a midwife to a more fortunate birth, a cosmic awakening like that achieved through traditional initiation in the mystery traditions. If jade is the stone that accompanies us to our deaths, then lapis prepares us for the next stage in our evolution. Jade is the stone of the shaman's death, the death of the ego, through which we can interact with our immortal self. Lapis, then, anchors the process of rebirth after this death.

It is said in some traditions that between incarnations the soul returns to the heavens in order to reflect on every experience and decide the path of the next incarnation. This return to the realm of the stars is the primal return to the womb of the Cosmic Mother for regeneration and resurrection. Lapis lazuli catalyzes the process of rebirth, and it guides the shamanic initiate into rebirth as the sage of his or her people.

The purpose of the journey across the heavens, like the scarab's mythical solar trek, is to know and reclaim our connection to Source before rebirth. Because humankind is descended from the stars, it is necessary to open our hearts to the vastness of space in order to own our heritage to its fullest extent. Lapis serves as a tool to shift our fundamental perception of the world to a heart-centered experience rather than being purely mental. Meditating with lapis lazuli can offer profound spiritual experiences, and that is why it is a stone that endures through the ages.

Through the process of the shaman's death and resurrection, the spiritual initiate is offered a unique perspective from the abode of the gods. The liminal, in-between state is the ideal setting for karmic healing, and lapis is one of the earth's best gems for releasing the trauma of karmic ties from this lifetime and beyond. While the soul travels to the heavens, new sight is granted, and as we are reborn we are given the gift of all-seeing eyes.

LAPIS LAZULI AS AN ARCHETYPE: THE ALL-SEEING EYE

Lapis lazuli has a longstanding association with the eyes and vision. Ancient texts indicate that it was valued as a restorative agent for failing eyesight and a panacea for disorders of the eyes. Throughout history, the calming, celestial color of lapis has been used for both healing and for beautifying the eyes, in the use of cosmetics and in art. This points to the second archetype of lapis lazuli: the all-seeing eye.

The all-seeing eye of God has been known by many names. To the people of ancient Egypt it was both the Eye of Horus and the Eye of Ra. Early Christian cultures fashioned this symbol as the Eye of Providence, which was transplanted in Freemasonry and other mystery traditions of the western world (see below). The all-seeing eye symbolizes the eye of the Creator looking out from the heavens on all of creation. Naturally, a gemstone that resembles the firmament above makes the ideal medium into which this sacred symbol can be carved.

Eyes represent vision and insight, both in the material and immaterial planes. Eyes are protective symbols, for they are watchful and can see evil coming. Poetically, they are also the windows to the soul, an opening to the internal workings of one's being. The watchful eye of God offers all of these capabilities, as well as providing a two-way connection to the heavenly realm.

The Evil Eye

As a protective charm, the eye is customarily thought to ward off evil and negativity in two ways: it is both watchful and attentive, therefore able to warn the wearer of a negative influence that is on its way. The Eye of Horus and the eyes of the Buddha are excellent examples of the watchful eyes of heavenly beings used for guidance and protection. On the other hand, charms and amulets representative of the evil eye are widespread; they offer protection by means of sympathetic resonance, which is based on the principle of "like attracts like." The evil eye is a curse common to many cultures; it is believed to originate with a malevolent gaze, and the recipient is generally unaware of its source. This curse is traditionally believed to bring harm or misfortune, and it is mitigated by small eye-shaped charms, also called evil eyes. These charms, often made of blue and white glass, function like homeopathic cures for the negative energy inherent in the curse.

Especially in the Middle East, evil eyes made of blue and white glass or ceramic are worn as amulets to avert the evil eye and other ills directed at one. Not only do these eyes watch over their wearers, they offer additional protection because their form as an eye works by means of sympathetic resonance to ward off the evil eye—the principle of "like cures like." It has been suggested that the color of these talismans is representative of lapis lazuli. Lapis has long been considered as warding off the evil eye because of its heavenly color, for evil cannot exist in the presence of the heavens. Writer and historian Sarah Searight suggests that the blue glass discs made to avert the evil eye are "an imitation of lapis lazuli" and are widely used to ensure safe travel.[15]

The evil eye is thought to stem from greed and attachment. When someone casts a scornful glance at another's prized possessions or looks on the success of another person without compassion, the negativity cast by their eyes is believed to be capable of acting like a curse. Essentially, the fundamental principle behind the evil eye is the attachment and suffering that accompanies it. Lapis lazuli appeals to spirit not only in turning away the negative effects of the evil eye, but it also grants hope and inspires a peaceful atmosphere. The starry beauty of this metamorphic rock speaks to the opening of the heart center and reminds one of the true abundance that is available when we remember our union with Creator.

While lapis lazuli may have been supplanted by ultramarine-colored glass in fashioning evil-eye amulets because of the cost and relative scarcity of lapis, the depiction of the eye in lapis's distinctive color remains to this day a testament to the tradition of lapis's protective qualities. Lapis lazuli awakens vision beyond just offering another set of vigilant eyes; it brings our awareness to a deeper level, by uniting our hearts and minds, which can enable us to see with the eyes of God.

The Eye of Horus

Horus is often depicted as a falcon or as a man with a falcon head. Falcons are birds of prey that soar to great heights. From their perspective in the heavens, birds of prey can survey all of creation below them. These raptors offer their "bird's eye view" when we connect to them spiritually, which is one of the uses of the Eye of Horus, or udjat (also known as the *wedjat*). Worship of sky deities through the use of the falcon is the earliest evidence of Egyptian religious culture. Similarly, the Eye of Horus is the world's first recorded incarnation of the all-seeing eye. The symbol is traditionally used to accompany the embalmed bodies of the deceased into the underworld, as well as to offer new vision to devotees who wear it in life.

Each of Horus's eyes was connected to a separate luminary; one represents the sun, while the other is sometimes representative of the moon. The overt solar imagery of the disclike form of the central part of the eye is not unlike the solar orb pushed along the sky by the divine scarab, and because of this, the two symbols are sometimes found in association with each other.

One of the most important spells found in the Egyptian Book of the Dead consists of the "form of an eye, fashioned out of lapis-lazuli and ornamented with gold"; it was believed to be an "amulet of great power."[16] This particular passage provides instructions for the construction of an amulet such as that worn by the supreme deity, Ra. From this it can be surmised that the holy eye was indeed one of Egypt's most important icons. The Egyptian mystery cults adapted the Eye of Horus into many uses and allowed its form to evolve into other sacred symbols. It is believed that the eye was used to express fractions and to calculate the complex mathematics needed for building the many sacred sites in Egypt. The form would eventually take on an overtly solar appearance that would later give rise to the Uraeus, the disc-shaped solar image flanked by one or more serpents, used as a symbol of sovereignty, royalty, deity, and divine authority in ancient Egypt. The artisans among ancient Egypt's dynasties used pigments made from lapis to depict the eyes of sacred beings, and even made eyes of lapis lazuli inset in wooden statues, too.[17] Famously, Egypt's distinctive cosmetics meant to be applied around the eyes were made of ground lapis. These not only looked quite striking on the eyes of those who wore this make-up, they surely must have also been used to grant spiritual vision and psychic insight to the wearers.

The Eye of Providence

The cryptic image of the Eye of Providence has worked its way into churches, seals, and onto U.S. currency. The eye, often contained within a pyramid or triangle, is meant to be a depiction of the all-seeing eye of God. The Eye of Providence contained within a pyramid, thus establishing a link to the ancient Egyptians, was preceded by the many ancient statues of deities whose eyes are carved from lapis lazuli as a testament to their heavenly, omniscient vision. Examples include the golden idol of Sin, the lunar god of Babylon, as well as an ancient goddess figure carved of ivory with inset lapis resembling sunglasses; while the lapis was likely a later addition to the statue, it nevertheless is said to resemble "the inlaid eyes such as have been found on devotional figures excavated at Tel el-Farkha in the Delta" of the Nile.[18]

The watchful Eye of Providence is an emblem of divine guidance and the vigilance that Creator has over creation. Lapis lazuli makes a perfect choice for conveying this concept in stone because of its pedigreed connection with the eyes and vision. Not only can it heal physical sight and correct illnesses of the eyes, lapis lazuli is prized as one of the stones par excellence for psychic vision. In today's tradition of using gemstones for healing, lapis lazuli is accepted as one of the best stones for opening the brow, or third-eye, chakra, which is located between and slightly above the eyebrows and is associated with functions of the higher mind and with intuitive pursuits of all types. The brow chakra is traditionally associated with the color indigo, although many crystal therapists also use violet and purple gems at the brow. The domain of the unknown, the spiritual, and the intuitive are all given to this particular energy center within our being. The stones most commonly used to promote the proper function of the third eye tend to be associated with intuition, telepathy, wisdom, spiritual growth, and knowledge.

Lapis, as a stone of the third eye, is best known for its ability to access the inner vision, thereby yielding self-knowledge. When the art of looking critically at ourselves is mastered, such as that which obsidian facilitates, then we can remove the masks we wear via jade, to penetrate even the darkest and most hidden mysteries of life. Lapis affects both the heart and the third eye, for they both represent our means of perceiving and processing the world around us—one emotionally, the other mentally and psychically.

Statues with lapis eyes, funeral masks with lapis brows, and even lapis eye paint clearly indicate its use for awakening a new type of vision beyond the mere material level of seeing. Lapis is both spiritually expansive, by reminding us to move upward into the heavens, as well as reductive, for it narrows the attention inward. No matter which direction you follow with lapis, in or out, it shows you that ultimately the same truth is revealed. You can follow the path of the soul out among the stars, or into the heart, and the same scenes can be experienced.

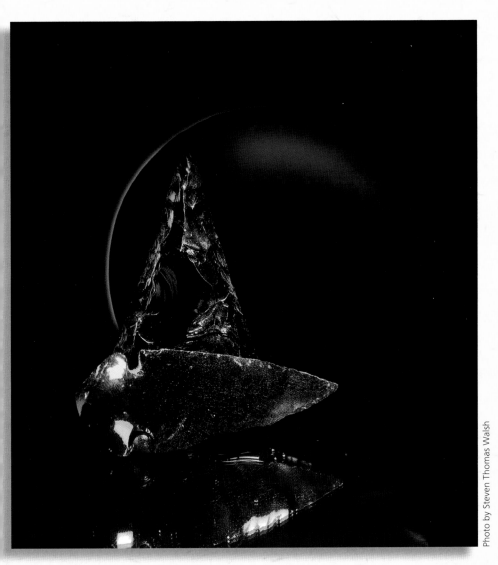

Plate 1. Obsidian
Arrowheads and polished mirror representing obsidian's archetypes

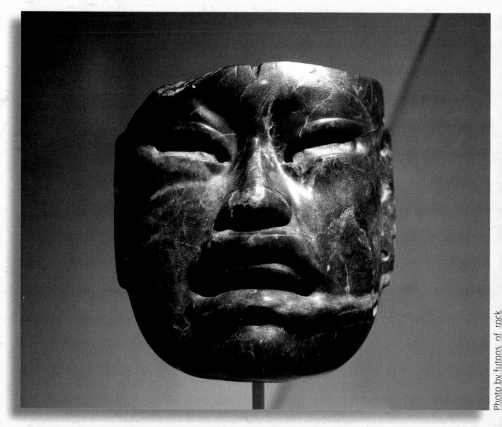

Plate 2. Jade
Olmec jadeite mask, 10th–6th century BCE, 6¾ x 6⁵⁄₁₆ x 6⁵⁄₁₆ inches,
Metropolitan Museum of Art, New York

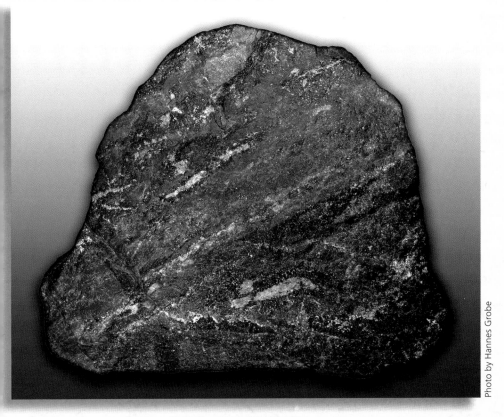

Plate 3. Lapis lazuli
Rough lapis lazuli from Badakhshan, Afghanistan

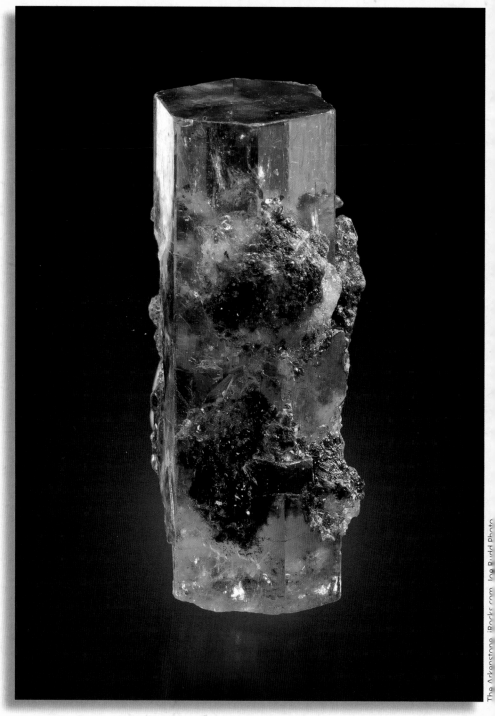

Plate 4. Emerald
Hexagonal crystal of emerald

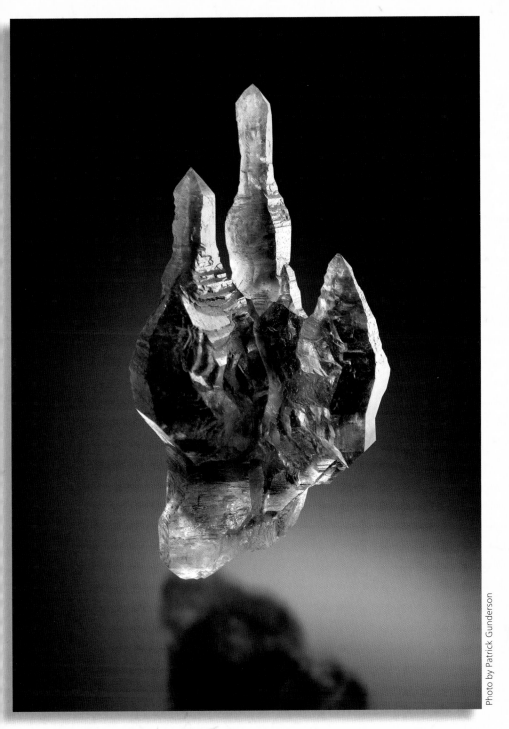

Plate 5. Amethyst
This Australian amethyst resembles a violet flame or a crystalline cathedral.

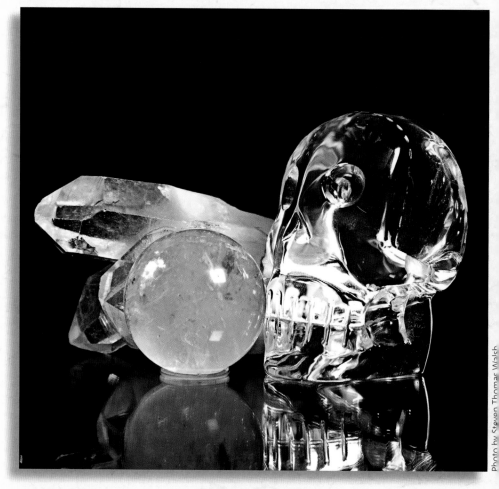

Plate 6. Quartz
A natural wand, polished sphere,
and crystal skull illustrate quartz's archetypes.

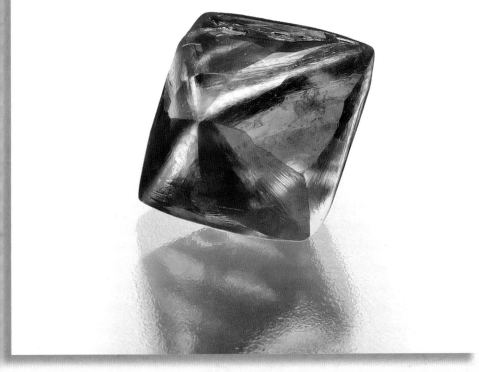

Plate 7. Diamond
Diamond's octahedral crystal forms are a
perfect symbol of the axiom "as above, so below."

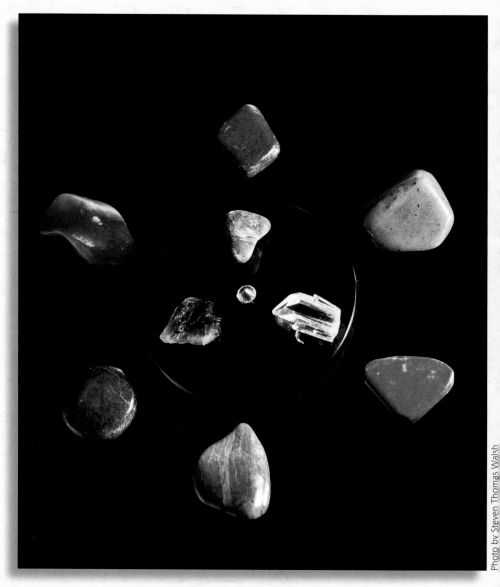

Plate 8. Crystal grid

A crystal grid made from the seven archetypal stones, consisting of
an outer ring of alternating jade and lapis lazuli; an inner ring of emerald,
amethyst, and quartz atop an obsidian mirror; and faceted diamond at the center.

The Mental Connection

The starry skies awaken the longing within our hearts, but lapis lazuli also stirs the mind into a state of awareness. The human eye is directly connected to the brain, and it provides much of the sensory information by which the environment is constantly being assessed by the mind. Eyes are expressive; they assist in our communication of ideas, concepts, and feelings. Lapis lazuli is a stone that bridges both the heart and the mind, for its energy acts as a pathway between the third eye and the heart centers, thereby facilitating communication and exchange between the two.

Blue stones are often associated with the mental functions of our being, from dissolving repetitive thoughts to uplifting one's outlook on life. Lapis serves as an incredible healer of the mental body because the hope it inspires displaces worry and fear. It also allows one to gaze at any thought form and see it for what it truly is, without having an emotional reaction to it. Best of all, lapis serves humanity by uniting the mind and the heart toward a common goal. Gemstone therapist Michael Katz writes, "Lapis Lazuli harmonizes your heart and mind as it forges stronger bonds between them. When your mind is attuned to your emotions, it is enriched and made more fruitful; when your emotions are illuminated by your mind, they become more clearly understood. With heart and mind working in harmony, mastery of any area of life becomes more attainable."[19]

The idea of unification is one of the basic properties of lapis lazuli. The Japanese view mind and heart as inherently inseparable, and they use the word *kokoro* (心) to indicate this concept. The idea of a unified heart-mind field is central to the role of lapis because it helps to heal the rift of perceiving separation on all levels, such as the separation between heart and mind, or between Creator and created. As this connection between the head and the heart is strengthened, it becomes a natural extension of their interrelationship to better express ideas and emotions. Lapis lazuli, as we shall soon learn, is also associated with the throat chakra, which marks the midway point between the heart and the third eye, thereby underscoring its action of uniting heart and mind.

MEDITATION
___

ACTIVATING THE ALL-SEEING EYE

A smallish, flat piece of lapis is preferred during this meditation. A tumbled stone or cabochon may be exactly the right fit, as it will lie on your forehead for the duration of this exercise. Lie down comfortably and have your lapis lazuli handy.

Begin by holding the stone to your heart. Imagine breathing in through the stone; as the breath passes through the stone and into the heart, it awakens and aligns with the heart chakra. Repeat this breathing pattern several times. When your heart is fully awakened, move the stone to your brow. Visualize yourself breathing in through the stone, just as before. As you inhale, it fills your third-eye chakra, awakening and aligning this energy center. Let this light permeate your entire head. As your third eye grows brighter, so does your heart; now they work in unison.

Continue to hold the visualization of your heart and third-eye chakras gleaming brightly, activated and harmonized by lapis lazuli. Each in-breath feeds these energy centers, and each out-breath exits through the throat chakra, clearing it and aligning it with the heart and third eye.

When you are ready to complete the meditation, remove the lapis lazuli from your brow and return it to your heart. Breathe gently and deeply, allowing any excess energy to flow through you and into the earth. Return your awareness to the room and open your eyes.

LAPIS LAZULI AS AN ARCHETYPE: THE WORD

For many, blue stones are related to the throat chakra and are associated with self-expression, communication, and truth. Lapis, being a stone of the throat chakra as well as the third eye, is used to heal not only the everyday forms of communication but also to express the archetypal word, as in the Word of God. Scriptural references to lapis lazuli stone tablets, illuminated manuscripts graced with ultramarine pigment, and lapis amulets and talismans inscribed with holy names and magical formulae illustrate the stone of heaven's connection to this archetype.

As we know, the intrinsic allure of lapis stems from its vibrant color and striking appearance. Harnessing the powers of the heavens was of utmost importance to ancient cultures such as that of Greece, and lapis lazuli endowed them with this ability. Early carvings of lapis include cylindrical seals bearing the names of their owners inscribed on them. While any stone could suffice for such a use, the lapis seals were especially prized because of their mystical properties. Using a lapis seal to sign a document would imbue the signature with the power of the heavens, thereby acting like the Word of God. Many such seals have been found in Knossos, a Bronze Age archeological site on the island of Crete; they denote the sovereignty of their bearers and the authority of their decrees.

Mughal aristocrats also favored lapis for inscribing with sacred words, such as the names and titles of Allah and the prophets. Protective amulets, known as *tughra,* feature prayerlike inscriptions that offer the grace of God to their bearers, and it is not uncommon to find these made of lapis. These carvings are vestiges of earlier uses of lapis that withstood the changing eras and became anchored in the Islamic world. The Koran is often found decorated with lavish geometric sketches in ultramarine pigments derived from lapis lazuli.

Later uses of lapis lazuli include the distinctive illuminated manuscripts of holy texts that appeared during the Middle Ages. Medieval religious writings and hand-copied Bibles often contain ornate details and lettering featuring lapis pigments. Sarah Searight writes, "On the whole lapis lazuli is reserved for the holiest biblical characters."[20]

The Tablets of the Law

In the context of language, both spoken and written, lapis lazuli is the archetype of the divine word, the law of God. "The sacred character of the stone was attested by the tradition that the Law given to Moses on the Mount was engraved on tablets of sapphire"; properly translated, this actually refers to lapis lazuli,[21] as sapphire was neither found in suitable sizes for engraved tablets nor easy to carve given the lapidary tools available in Moses's time. These engraved tablets contained the Ten Commandments, considered the Word of God. Lapis lazuli, here called *sappir* in Hebrew, was chosen because it is indicative of the sovereignty of the Heavenly Father and the holiness of his word. The commandments were written in lapis because it made manifest the very law of the heavens and radiated this to all who gazed at the tablets.

Other sacred tablets of lapis exist in history and myth. Nisaba, the Sumerian goddess of writing, accounting, and grain, owned her own sacred engraving. "Lapis is the stone used for the Tablet of the Stars of the Heavens," and it may have been the stone on which she chronicled all history and kept the accounts of Creation.[22] Nisaba is credited as the inventor of writing and is a master teacher, having instructed both mortal and godly scribes in her arts.

The efficacy and function of lapis is intimately associated with the power of the word and its ability, whether spoken or written, to manifest physical reality. The biblical Creation account shows that God spoke the heavens and earth into existence. The first exclamation was "Let there be Light," and there was light; God's power to create stems from his use of the word. In John 1:1 we read, "In the beginning was the Word, and the Word was with God, and the Word was God."

Lapis engravings, seals, and pigments are a palpable example of the ability to manifest through the archetypal word. With any of these uses of lapis lazuli, the word is literally made manifest; the word can be seen and felt, rather than merely comprehended on a mental level. Lapis empowers the word to create from the heavenly realms and be made manifest in physical reality. This is the alchemical process of taking the implicate order of the universe, that which cannot be seen or experienced with the physical senses, and creating something explicate and influential in the three-dimensional world that we experience.

Alchemy of the Word

Ultramarine pigment was used for accenting consecrated icons and illuminating hallowed scripture. The term *ultramarine* is derived from the Latin *ultramarinus,* literally "beyond the sea," because the pigment was imported into Europe from mines in Afghanistan by Italian traders during the fourteenth and fifteenth centuries. This title is bestowed also for ultramarine's depth of color, being bluer than seawater. Lapis lazuli serves as the basis for this expensive pigment. The process of extracting the blue powder from host rock resembles alchemy, not unlike the inner alchemy required to achieve spiritual mastery through the use of lapis in meditative pursuits.

Alchemy, the process of transmutation of a base material into a more rarefied form, is an excellent metaphor for spiritual progress. Medieval alchemists rose to fame for pursuing the legendary philosopher's stone, a substance that was believed would transform lead into gold and could be used to distill the elixir of life, which granted immortality. Alchemists perfected their arts and mastered the elements in order to achieve this goal, known as the Great Work. Though a discussion of alchemy is beyond the scope of this book, it can be said that the alchemical arts represent the rarefaction of the human spirit through mastery over the elements and the processes of our unfolding being.

To produce a good ultramarine pigment, pounds and pounds of the finest lapis lazuli must be ground and sifted into a fine powder. It is then mixed with resins or oils and wax to produce a kneadable dough. The blue color is then extracted in a caustic solution and dried. It can then be mixed with water, egg, or another medium in order to be used as paint. In this arduous process very little usable powder results from the initial large quantities of raw material.

This act of separation and gradual refinement is not unlike the actions undertaken in alchemy. The separation of "the elements of lapis lazuli—lazurite, calcite and iron pyrites—related to the four elements that so absorbed medieval alchemists. Lazurite represents air, calcite water, earth iron pyrites, and fire fuses all three."[23] Alchemists use the natural elements and refine them in order to effect change in the world. Lapis helps us gain our own sense of mastery to create our reality with the tools at our disposal—chiefly, the power of the word.

Ultramarine pigment has as its most sanctified use the illumination of the Word of God. Even the art of illumination takes its name from the idea of light; this light represents spiritual power, the power to create. God's first decree in the act of Creation was the moment in which light was created and separated from darkness. Reading antiquated manuscripts with illuminated letters calls forth the power of the gemstones used to thus illumine the mind. Speaking them aloud engenders within one the power to create. Lapis lazuli's connection to the power of the spoken word goes back to ancient Egypt. The twenty-sixth chapter of the Egyptian Book of the Dead contains an incantation that must be recited before a figure of carved lapis in order to obtain the desired result.[24]

Sacred letters are first read with the eyes; the characters are then interpreted by the brain and comprehended by the mind. From there, the Word of God is anchored in our hearts, such that we may act on it with proper intent. Together, heart and mind act as one to express the word. We see that lapis's function as a harmonizer of these two centers always results in the opening of expression, as the throat center that lies between the two is similarly aligned and opened. One who can use words in this way can be considered a poet. "A true bard, or spiritual master, makes words into vehicles of light, for his words are charged with a spiritual energy beyond that of ordinary language. Such words have the power to illumine those who can listen and truly hear."[25] Alchemy, therefore, is the process of raising our vibration in order to use the word with authentic mastery.

Sovereignty and Power

The distinctive shade of blue for which lapis is renowned is often referred to as "royal blue." In part this was because of the value placed on ultramarine pigment due to its great expense in mining, refining, and shipping across the world; only the wealthy could afford to commission sacred art that utilized this hue. Other pigments, such as the synthetically derived Egyptian blue, manufactured from silica sand, ash, and ores of copper, or the azure blue made from azurite were often used in place of ultramarine, with highlights of royal blue paint on top to give these substitutes depth. The wealthy classes and royalty soon became associated with this blue pigment made from lapis.

Lapis lazuli featured among crown jewels and scepters, both real and mythological. It made its place on signet rings and seals not only for being easily carved, but because it was thought to confer the sovereignty of the heavens over those who possessed such a precious gem. However, true power does not come from one's class or rank; power and mastery result from accessing the heavens that reside within the heart of humanity, the spark of divinity intrinsic to all life.

Even the mining of the gemstone of heaven requires mastery over the elements. In what is now Afghanistan, ancient miners trekked great distances to access remote mines in the mountains that are home to the finest lapis. "They would set a fire near the vein of lapis embedded in limestone, then after heating the area, douse it with cold water. Finally a pick would be used to chip out a vein of blue stone."[26] Fire, water, and earthy iron would be used to extract the raw stone reserved for royalty, and the process of distillation and refinement continued from there. It is necessary to have control over the very elements just to gain a rough piece of gem material; lapis lazuli is not a stone for the uninitiated.

Lapis comes to us to remind us of our inherent royal lineage. We are literally and figuratively descended from stardust. Creation myths from many cultures indicate that humankind comes from the heavens. In some, the Heavenly Father fashions us by his hand; in others we were birthed on this planet by races that dwell among the stars. Science even shows that we are comprised of the same matter once occupying the stars that formed all we see and know today.

When we accept our royal heritage from the Creator, we accept that we all have the power to rule our destinies. The unification of head and heart allows for a clear channel by which this power can be gathered. This sovereignty is channeled and expressed through the word, because once the intrinsic spark of the word is claimed, it is then possible to shape your reality and co-create with the universe. The word becomes law when we choose to operate from the state of spiritual mastery.

Healing Separation Consciousness

The fundamental lie our egos perceive is one of separation. It is the easiest illusion to buy into, especially if it is assessed as being two people who are discrete corporeal entities; they cannot occupy the same space and are clearly separate individuals. This perception fuels the idea of our separateness from one another, as well as from Source. The Judeo-Christian teachings describe the "fall from grace" first experienced in the Garden of Eden, and the subsequent punishment inflicted on humankind.

Lapis lazuli is a stone that visually calls to mind a clear image of the heavenly firmament, and yet the stone is undoubtedly a grounding, earthy rock. This celestial gemstone is a simple and powerful reminder that the earth is not separate from the heavens; the divine is omnipresent and can be experienced in all matter and energy within the universe. For this reason, we as human beings cannot be separate from the divine at any given moment or in any location. The only way to experience the illusion of separation is to forget the intrinsic unity in which we are created. This is what is really meant by the fall from grace, because it is by believing in our separateness from God that we lose our divinity.

Lapis lazuli, a starry stone of heavenly significance, brings the essence of the divine into the earthly realm. When held or meditated on it enlivens the spark of oneness within the person. Lapis lazuli grounds this right view of the interrelationship between the human and celestial kingdoms into the person's heart and mind, resulting in a new form of consciousness and perception. This shift from separation consciousness into unity consciousness is the foundation of all healing, spiritual growth, and planetary ascension.

This perceptual shift yields indescribable effects. It eliminates feelings of lack, because anyone who recognizes his or her indivisible place in God's creation cannot experience the lack of anything. Infinite abundance, love, and health are always available as our perfected human nature, and as spiritual leaders our role is to share this through the word. As the heart and mind are harmonized, the throat chakra becomes the medium through which unity consciousness can be expressed. Although we may not choose to do so through the spoken or written word, the presence of this frequency can be enough to initiate similar shifts in other people. In the eleventh century, one bishop, writing of lapis, said that it "signifies that those who are placed on earth aspire for heavenly things."[27]

Finding Your Seat on the Throne

The Book of Ezekiel (1:26) opens with a visitation from God to the Hebrew prophet Ezekiel, in which God appears on a chariot drawn by four fantastic beasts. Over this chariot God's throne is visible: "And over their heads was the likeness of a throne, in appearance like a sapphire stone." This ancient stone described as sapphire was really lapis lazuli, and it was chosen as the very throne of the Almighty. In addition to the throne of the Hebrew God, the Egyptian goddess Isis was also known by the epithet Throne of Horus, because Horus, her son, was often shown seated in her lap. Carvings of the divine mother and child are often rendered in lapis lazuli, thus cementing the choice of the stone of heaven to represent the throne of the sovereign of the celestial sphere.

Divine beings as well as kings and queens are traditionally depicted with ultramarine pigment. During the Middle Ages and the Renaissance, blue paints derived from lapis served as the preferred color for depicting the robes of the Madonna and Christ Child, as well as the haloes surrounding saints and other holy figures. In the Buddhist world, illustrations of bodhistattvas and buddhas on ancient cave murals are also artfully shown in robes of lapis or with lapis-colored skin. One particular buddha, the Medicine Buddha, is nearly always shown with skin a rich royal blue. The Medicine Buddha's moniker is "Medicine Master and King of Lapis Lazuli Light." Lapis lazuli is a stone reserved only for those who have had power and authority conferred on them from the highest power of Creator.

Lapis lazuli is a stone of spiritual mastery. Mastery occurs when heart and mind are working in total unity, with no separation. Likewise, spiritual teachers, leaders, and trailblazers are generally those who perceive no separation between humanity and the Source from which we all spring. Lapis lazuli helps one to grow to one's fullest potential by realizing this intrinsic spiritual connectedness; this is the most effective way to take on spiritual leadership during these times of transition on planet Earth.

Lapis lazuli is among the important stones featured in the Bible. It appears as the second foundation stone in New Jerusalem, as the throne in Ezekiel's vision, and as a stone in the breastplate of Aaron representing the tribe of Dan. "The selection of lapis as the second foundation stone is significant. The number two represents division or separation. The name Dan is defined in Hebrew as 'dawn, to judge, to rule.' The word sapphire [*cappiyr*] represents 'scratching, to score, inscribe . . . declare.'"[28] Even the color blue symbolizes a "reminder of Heaven and the authority we carry."[29] This exploration of the etymology of the word *lapis* and the history of lapis lazuli's biblical significance further expresses the power of the word and the sovereignty of those who express it as a quality of spiritual mastery.

MEDITATION

SITTING ON THE THRONE

You may select either a piece of lapis jewelry to wear or a stone to hold during this meditation. After it has been cleansed, hold the intention that the lapis will help you to reclaim your sovereignty. Place it in your hands or otherwise wear it as appropriate, and sit comfortably in order to begin the meditation.

Close your eyes and imagine that there is a beautiful building before you. It resembles something between a temple and a castle. A path is laid out clearly in front of you, and it leads directly to the entrance of the building. Follow it and enter this sacred space. Within, you come to a doorway that leads into an elaborate throne room. Directly opposite the doorway is an exquisite throne carved of lapis lazuli. Make your way across the room and sit on the throne.

As you sit, breathe deeply and evenly. With each in-breath visualize a royal blue light filling your being. Let it penetrate any patterns of unworthiness. Let it sink into the areas of your being where you do not feel as though you are in control. Let this light wash over you, granting you the authority and power to create the life that you want. As you breathe in the lapis lazuli light, your entire being vibrates to the same frequency. Picture yourself becoming a being of pure, lapis-colored brilliance. If any resistance arises, command it to kneel before your throne. Bless it, and send it on its way, for it no longer has control over you. Repeat this process any time that fear or unease makes itself known.

When you have completed this task, arise from your throne and return to your physical body. Breathe deeply and allow the energy of lapis lazuli to integrate you totally. When you are ready, open your eyes.

LAPIS LAZULI IN CRYSTAL HEALING

In the ancient world, lapis lazuli was prized for its curative and therapeutic properties. The ocular imagery associated with lapis overlaps with its primary use in many cultures for disorders of the eyes, but it is a supreme healer on all levels. Lapis is a powerful spiritual healer, for it is sacred to Bhaisajyaguru, the Medicine Buddha, whose epithet is "Medicine Master and Lord of the Lapis Lazuli Light." Temples devoted to the Medicine Buddha exist throughout the Buddhist world. He is the master healer and physician whose medicine is his teachings. In Buddhist cosmology the Medicine Buddha rules over the Eastern Paradise, a land of lapis lazuli.

The oldest extant writings about lapis lazuli connect its use to healing disorders of the eyes, head, inflammatory illness, and the stomach.

The soothing blue color of lapis was traditionally considered a balm for the eyes. Not only was it understood to enhance psychic vision, it was often applied to the eyes to restore eyesight. While the stone was occasionally placed directly on the eyes, it was more common to use water in which lapis had been soaked as an eyewash to heal one's vision. Placing tumbled pieces of lapis on the eyes may help alleviate the symptoms of eyestrain and promote general relaxation, too.

Structurally, the granular composition of this metamorphic rock resembles the retina, with its network of calcite veins and sodalite-group minerals suspended in a matrix like the rods and cones of the eyes. The sulfur found within its structure is closely associated with the nature of life itself, as sulfur "promotes the enlivening process of protein," and it may be excellent for combating degenerative disorders of the eyes.[30]

Lapis lazuli is also connected to the circulatory system, for it is found as veins in its host matrix. Ultramarine pigment also served as the ideal color for painting veins in Renaissance portraiture. Traditional as well as New Age sources report that lapis lazuli may promote the healing of blood disorders, and its positive effect may extend to lowering high blood pressure and reducing inflammation.[31] Since ancient times, lapis has been connected with the heart, both in a metaphorical and an anatomical sense, and for this reason it is recommended for heart diseases of all types.

The addition of pyrite and calcite to the overall effects of lapis lazuli render it an excellent stone for promoting general physical health and vitality. Pyrite, a cubic iron sulfide, is a natural semiconductor. As such it may help to promote the electrical conductivity of the nervous system, and its sulfur content may even support the repair of damaged nerve tissue. This is supported by the stone's association with the third-eye chakra, which often includes the nervous system.

In addition, both pyrite and calcite are excellent for offering structural support to our physical bodies. The cubic crystal system of pyrite as well as that of lazurite represents order, structure, and grounding.

The calcium content of calcite is also beneficial for the bones and teeth. On a deeper level, the indigo ray as described in gemstone therapy is related to form and structure, which are overtly Saturnian qualities. In healing, indigo-colored gems can be employed for improving physical form and supporting structural integrity, such as that of the skeletal system. Medical astrologers ascribe the skeletal system to Saturn's rule, and lapis is even associated with Saturn in ayurveda.[32] Taken together, lapis's unique composition offers excellent support on all levels of the physical makeup. Lapis lazuli is also recommended for the health of the throat and tonsils, the thymus gland, the thyroid, and for the assimilation of nutrients.[33]

As a mental-emotional healer, lapis lazuli truly shines. It helps to heal and uplift the spirits through the unification of heart and mind. This can lead to a better understanding of one's emotions and can heighten mental awareness overall.[34] Traditional sources connect lapis lazuli to a heavenly sense of hope, and the depth of color can provide inspiration where none can otherwise be found.

Lapis lazuli is one of my favorite stones to promote mental mastery. It can foster wisdom and understanding, as well as provide a healthy outlet for the expression of one's emotions. In ancient Greece and Rome, the stone of heaven was a popular choice to promote friendship and fidelity. It makes an exceptional stone for clarifying the emotions and allowing your voice to be heard. The emotional context of lapis is always tempered by the intellectual bridge it creates, thereby granting eloquence and grace in one's communication, so there is never any fear of misrepresenting one's thoughts or feelings.

The pyrite and calcite present in lapis help bolster its mental and emotional support. Calcite, as a rhombic mineral, embodies a crystalline geometry that expresses the connections between parallel realities. This is symbolized by the rhombus-shaped cleavage that calcite exhibits. Calcite can help one make better leaps in understanding, as well as to better connect the evidence at hand in any situation. Because it forms from an aqueous solution, it is also tempered to heal our emotional body; it does so by helping to release the fears and hurts garnered in childhood. Pyrite is an excellent stone for promoting logical thinking; the rigid, cubic lattice responsible for its morphology is a great aid to discipline and remaining level-headed.

As a stone of spiritual mastery, lapis lazuli brings spiritual healing to a deeper level than either obsidian or jade. Among all the gems prescribed by Edgar Cayce, lapis was held in highest esteem as a stone of spiritual healing. This stone promotes a level of wisdom and self-knowledge unparalleled by many other gems, and it ultimately awakens the inner psychic senses.

Lapis lazuli awakens the qualities of intuition, insight, and a sense of unbridled hope. It awakens the third-eye chakra and allows its wearer to connect to the wisdom carried by the very stars. It also promotes a heart-centered approach to spiritual endeavors; placing a piece of lapis lazuli on the heart center can enhance the process of manifestation by channeling love into the creative flow. It offers a "very spiritual, idealistic energy that is also down-to-earth and practical," and it can promote pragmatism along the spiritual path.[35]

As a stone for liberating the human spirit, lapis gives the self a bird's-eye view of life and the lessons of karma. "Lapis lazuli offers one the opportunity for a life review before death, allowing one to integrate one's experiences so one can move on to a higher level of awareness."[36] It is especially well-suited to resolving karma from Egyptian lifetimes, as well as connecting to the wisdom of the ancients who used this heavenly gem. It enhances the meditative state and allows the mind and heart to receive spiritual teachings unencumbered by the ego. Lapis is truly the stone of adeptness and mastery.

Varieties of Lapis Lazuli

Afghani Lapis

Lapis lazuli from Afghanistan is generally regarded as the most beautiful and valuable. Spiritually, because it forms in such a perfect shade of ultramarine, it captures the celestial essence of serenity, hope, and spiritual growth. All of the properties of lapis described in this chapter are perfectly exemplified by Afghani lapis.

Denim Lapis

This is the name given to lower-quality pieces of lapis in which the white is nearly equal to blue in its total makeup. Generally, it is applied to stones of Chilean origin. Denim lapis has an overall softer, more diffuse energy than richer, denser varieties of lapis. It can teach one to better listen to the needs of the body, making it a great stone for enhancing the abilities of medical intuitives. Denim lapis soothes tired limbs and is especially suited for use on long journeys. It provides stamina, presence, and protection along the way.

Lapis Diopside

An uncommon form, lapis diopside has a higher than usual quantity of diopside in its composition. Many times the diopside will have displaced calcite in its structure. This particular combination is very powerful for connecting to inner guidance and enhancing intuitive faculties. The additional diopside is strengthening and supportive. Diopside has a heavenly energy of its own, given that it is one of jade's constituent minerals, and so it lends the strength and tenacity of jade to lapis. It permits a deeper view into the inner workings of things, and this brings a logical slant to the intuitive nature of lapis lazuli.

Pakistani Lapis

Lapis lazuli from Pakistan is a new addition to my crystal toolbox. The pieces that I have seen are generally a deep indigo, and they are streaked with very little calcite and solid veins of pyrite. Like lapis from other locations, the quality can vary quite a bit, and no two pieces are alike. Generally, I have found that this variety of lapis is more grounding than others. It perfectly expresses the indigo ray and is an optimal stone for tapping into the energies and ideals of Saturn. Like the ringed planet,

Pakistani lapis is associated especially with learning karmic lessons. It helps us to see why we reap what we have sown.

Pakistani lapis is an excellent stone for teachers; it can help one to effectively communicate lessons and ensure that students do not get lost. Lapis lazuli from Pakistan is a good choice for anyone who has difficulty breaking down complex concepts for others; it helps the mind to more effectively comprehend the pieces and to express them in simple, meaningful terms.

Related Stones

Azurite

Azurite shares a linguistic root with lapis lazuli; it, too, is derived from the Persian root word that describes its deep blue color. Azurite is a carbonate of copper and was the original source for the blue pigment azure, which though deep, lacks the brilliance and translucency of ultramarine pigment. Azurite shares lapis's association with the third eye, and it provides enhanced perception and insight. Azurite's copper component aids in exploring matters related to the emotions, as well as providing malleability and conductivity to its energy.

Azurite "gives the ability to 'read between the lines' in what others would have us believe," which in turn makes it a great stone for uncovering the truth and sharpening discernment.[37] It empowers the mind to sharpen its focus, and it is "a helpful aid for those who are studying new and challenging subjects."[38] Azurite may also enhance psychic pursuits and allow one to shield oneself, thus practicing the art of invisibility.

K2

K2 is the name for a newly available type of granite. It is currently mined in Pakistan, in the foothills of the world's second-highest peak, from which this stone derives its name. It is comprised of quartz, feldspar, biotite mica, and splotches of royal blue that are believed to be azurite. The translucent patches of blue stand out against the otherwise plainly colored background. Granite is an intrusive igneous rock, and it is supremely grounding and nurturing. It consists of a cocktail of mostly silicate minerals that can enliven and root us in the earth. The intensely blue patches of azurite represent a more rarefied and celestial vibration, thus enabling this stone to effectively bridge heaven and earth, not unlike lapis lazuli.

K2 is still relatively unexplored energetically. My own experiences with this stone show me that it teaches about solitude and serenity. Meditating with K2 is an experience like retreating to a mountain cave and seeking sanctuary away from the world. It can alleviate feelings of loneliness when one is isolated and trains the mind to be more present. K2 strengthens your entire being and promotes resiliency in the face of the everyday trials we face. Like other forms of granite, it can be protective, especially with regard to negative thoughts. K2 helps one to be less susceptible to the inner thoughts that are damaging, and it helps one to claim power and celebrate personal growth with grace.

Pyrite

Pyrite, sometimes referred to as "fool's gold," is the metallic-colored component of lapis lazuli's metamorphic structure. As the limestone matrix is gradually transformed, some of the sulfur is bound to iron, and this provides the sidereal sparkle that graces this celestial gem. Pyrite is masculine and grounding; its name is derived from the sparks that are produced when it is struck. It acts as the catalyst for inspiration, sparking new ideas and grounding them into the physical plane.

Pyrite on its own is often used to attract luck and wealth. Easily confused for more precious mineral treasures by inexperienced miners, pyrite helps one to question the true worth of any situation. It reminds you to look past material wealth to find that which is spiritually abundant behind the glittery veil of the three-dimensional world. Pyrite is grounding and supportive, but its iron content connects it to the warlike planet Mars. Because of this, it incites action and prevents stagnation. Pyrite is an excellent partner for lapis lazuli, especially if the frequency of lapis feels too grave or serious.

Sapphire

A variety of corundum, this aluminum oxide may come in any color except red. Blue sapphires are the most famous, and red corundum is known as another gemstone, ruby. Sapphire is worth being addressed here even if just for the shared name and history; ancient inscriptions and medieval lapidaries all call lapis lazuli "sapphire" by one means or another. For this reason, many of the qualities of lapis lazuli have been attributed to sapphire since antiquity.

Sapphire is prized for its transparency, hardness, and true blue color. It is an excellent mental healer, for it purifies the mental bodies and clears thought patterns at their most fundamental level. Sapphire is also recognized for providing strength of mind, willpower, and determination in all pursuits. Older sources attribute the same sense of celestial hope that lapis embodies to this blue stone, and it is a crystal that may be harnessed for clarity of focus, too.

Sodalite

Sodalite is actually the name of a class of minerals characterized by very similar compositions and cubic crystal structures. Lazurite is among the sodalite group, as are hackmanite, hauyne, and nosean. Sodalite's name is derived from the metal sodium, one of its primary components and the source of its dark blue color.

Sodalite is a stone of communication and connection. It can bring the mind into a greater sense of awareness, and it also engenders better communication. Sodalite is one of the chief stones for the throat chakra, although the dark blue to indigo color is sometimes prescribed for use at the third eye as well. Sodalite makes communication not only easier on behalf of the speaker, like most throat chakra stones, it also deepens the connection during communication to benefit the listener as well. This principle is applicable for other means of communication too. It may even aid animal communication and heighten psychic receptivity for connecting with nonphysical beings. Gemlike, crystalline sodalite is among the premier stones for building trust in one's intuition.

Sodalite from the Princess Mine in Bancroft, Canada, is an especially potent form of the mineral. It often contains unusual accessory minerals, including hackmanite, cancrinite, nepheline, and occasionally pyrite, among others. It conveys a very electric feeling and helps clear and align the energy pathways of the body. It is both earthy and spiritually expansive, which enables it to facilitate communication interpersonally and spiritually.

Hauyne

Hauyne, or hauynite, is a specific member of the sodalite group, and it is actually the parent mineral of which lazurite, lapis lazuli's chief constituent, is a subvariety. Gem-quality hauyne is a transparent, electric blue crystal, and it is considered to be one of the world's rarest gemstones. Large specimens are rarely found, thus making faceted stones of any considerable size nearly impossible to find. Its color associates this stone with the Virgin Mary; the ultramarine pigment used to paint her mantle is derived from its close relative, lapis lazuli.

Hauyne heals the feminine side of both men and women. It imparts a sense of returning to innocence without naivete. It "teaches that we can give with a free heart. We are perpetually receiving blessings. Giving and taking is a cycle; the one is dependent on the other."[39] One of the central messages of this diminutive blue stone is resurrection, for it helps us to "begin anew in every moment."[40]

White Calcite

Calcite is perhaps the most underappreciated element in lapis lazuli. The most exceptional specimens of lapis should have little-to-no visible calcite, but without calcite there is no lapis. Calcite acts as the glue that binds together the microscopic particles of blue crystals in the mass that is recognized as lapis lazuli. Therefore, even entirely blue pieces of lapis are not calcite-free.

Calcite is a carbonate of calcium, and it is one of nature's most versatile minerals. Calcite may be found in every color imaginable, and the variety of crystal forms is myriad. Mineral collectors around the globe specialize in calcites because of their unending diversity and beauty. White calcite, though arguably one of the commoner colors, is not without merit. It makes an excellent tool for providing mental acuity, and inclusion-free specimens will demonstrate the property of double refraction. This optical effect produces a double image of anything placed beneath the calcite.

The doubly refractive nature of calcite acts as a teacher who shows what it is like from every perspective in a given situation. White calcite is a soft stone that forms from the action of solution and chemical sedimentation. The close relationship that calcite has with water grants a watery, emotional quality to the essence of calcite, and it helps develop empathy and compassion when used consciously. Calcite is a great all-purpose stone and can be applied to virtually any situation for a variety of intended outcomes.

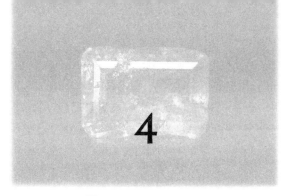

EMERALD

The Grail and the Tablet

As green as the most serene garden, emerald is a gemstone treasured above many others. Emerald has been valued throughout history for its color and rarity. It is a precious gem, considered to be the pinnacle of the "big four" gemstones: diamond, emerald, sapphire, and ruby. Emeralds have been mined and traded since ancient Egyptian times, and they have beguiled rulers, merchants, holy men, and the laity for millennia. Emeralds are sought after for their intriguing hue, which evokes images of fertile forests, and for their luminous brilliance that shines like the morning star at twilight.

Emerald is a variety of beryl. As such, it is an aluminum beryllium silicate, and its color is derived largely from trace amounts of chromium and vanadium. Beryls of other colors are also used as gemstones, including aquamarine (blue to green), goshenite (colorless), heliodor (golden to greenish yellow), morganite (pink), and bixbite (deep red). Varying amounts of trace elements grant each variety of beryl its appropriate range of colors. In the case of emerald, its green color is due to the presence of chromium, although vanadium has also been determined to yield a suitably green gem.

Emerald is formed under conditions of great heat and pressure as a result of several processes within the earth, largely metamorphic and igneous in nature. Beryl owes its unique properties to its eponymous element, beryllium. Beryllium is a relatively unstable element on its own; it has a short life span when synthesized in stars, and it virtually never occurs as an isolated element in nature. Accordingly, it is very rare in Earth's crust, constituting only 1.5 parts per million. The addition of chromium does not ordinarily occur where beryllium forms as part of minerals, thus contributing to the scarcity of emeralds on the earth.

Beryl, and therefore emerald, is a hexagonal mineral. Its crystal form is usually prismatic, forming six-sided columnar shapes. In belonging to the hexagonal crystal system, emeralds have four axes, and they display great amounts of symmetry in their idealized forms. Gem-quality emeralds are typically small, with larger stones often heavily marked by imperfections. In fact, of any precious gemstone, only emerald is considered to be acceptable even with visible flaws.

The flaws inherent to most emeralds may be the result of inclusions of solids, liquids, or gases; they may also be due to stress fractures incurred either during the gem's time in the earth or from its mining. The abundance and specific form that these inclusions take provide clues to the origin of any emerald, and can be used like fingerprints to identify their source. These inclusions may take the form of abstract, plantlike structures called *jardin,* French for "garden," in the gemstone industry.

Variations in the shades of green in an emerald are the result of how much chromium is present in the composition of beryl. Chromium substitutes for the aluminum in its crystal lattice, although iron and vanadium may be present too. Those stones colored by chromium alone tend to be a true emerald green, with undertones of yellow. Those with iron present have a visibly darker, bluer shade of green. Vanadium-bearing emeralds have a grayish cast and were only accepted as true emeralds by the gem trade in the United States after their discovery in Brazil in the 1970s. Exact shades of natural stones vary significantly, providing collectors with numerous options to suit personal preferences. The gemstone industry regularly treats emeralds. Cracks and fissures in their structure may be filled with oils and other substances, sometimes with dye added to them to improve their color. The practice of enhancing emeralds is as old as their provenance in ancient Egypt, although most practitioners of the spiritual arts favor untreated gems.

Emeralds may be found in many locations worldwide, though few yield commercially viable amounts and qualities suitable for the gemstone industry. Colombia is considered to be the world's leader in emerald production for the fine quality of stones it produces. Other locations where emeralds are found include Zambia, Zimbabwe, Australia, Canada, Afghanistan, Pakistan, Brazil, Bulgaria, Russia, the United States, India, and Egypt. A number of other locations also produce minor amounts of this green gem. Each location produces a stone with a unique makeup, including the constituent elements that provide the gems their exact hue. Because of this, trained gemologists are able to discern the origin of natural stones upon inspection.

Emerald owes its name to a Greek word *smaragdos,* which once referred to any green stone. This linguistic root can be traced through the Latin *smaragdus* into the English *emerald* via Old French and, further back, vulgar Latin. While the word once constituted an umbrella term for any green gem (much like *sapphirus* indicates virtually all blue stones), it was at times accurately applied to the beryl that we know as emerald.

EMERALD LORE

Emerald has served as the inspiration for many myths throughout human history. The fabled green gem of myth and legend is often imbued with magical properties, allowing it to persist and transform through the eons. Indigenous cultures of South America attribute the origin of emeralds to the earliest members of the human race. In the Muzo tribe of Colombia, emeralds were believed to originate from the tears of the first woman, who lived in a proverbial paradise not unlike Eden.

The Inca considered the green stone a sacred object to their Mother Goddess, Umiña; all emeralds were considered her children.

In the Old World, the mythic origin of emeralds can be traced to the heavens. Before the creation of humankind, the most precious of all emeralds adorned the crown of Lucifer, God's favored angel. However, when his rebellion against God resulted in him being cast out of heaven, Lucifer's emerald fell out of the diadem that graced his head. This very emerald was rumored to be in the treasury of the Queen of Sheba, and it was thought by some to be carved later into the Holy Grail itself.

In Islamic cultures the verdant shade of emerald was attributed to paradise, and it was regarded as a heavenly stone. Muslims preserved an Egyptian myth in which an emerald was carved into a sacred tablet bearing holy words; the Koran itself is said to have an earlier version carved in stone, called the "Mother of the Book." This representation of an emerald tablet influenced not only the Middle East but also the alchemical lore of Europe, as its mythic origins and mysterious content intrigued ancient scholars in many nations.

Traditionally, emerald was considered to have a healing influence over the eyes as well as the ability to cure cases of poisoning and protect against the bites of serpents and other venomous creatures. It was thought to inspire fidelity and encourage a pure, unconditional love, as well as to grant long life and serenity to its owner. Emerald is a gem whose healing virtues persist into the present, as it is believed to be an excellent tool for seeking the truth, attaining physical health, and healing emotional burdens.

EMERALD AS AN ARCHETYPE: THE EMERALD TABLET

The lore around emeralds include a number of tales referring to a certain green tablet on which are inscribed instructions for performing the Great Work of the alchemical arts. This tablet is described as being made of emerald. In some tales it is said to have been poured into a mold while in a molten state, while others describe it as having been carved or etched with the secrets of the universe on its surface. In any case, a cryptic piece of the *Hermetica,* an Egyptian-Greek wisdom text dating from around the second to third century CE, reputed to contain the secret of the *prima materia* and its transmutation, is a tract titled the *Emerald Tablet,* also known as the *Smaragdine Table,* or *Tabula Smaragdina.* The original source of the *Emerald Tablet* is unknown, although Hermes Trismegistus is the author named in the text. The first known appearance of this text is in a book written in Arabic between the sixth and eighth centuries. It was translated into Latin in the twelfth century, and numerous translations, interpretations, and commentaries followed, including one by Sir Isaac Newton.

While the existence of such a magical emerald tablet is largely relegated to the world of myth, throughout history the gem trade has been inspired by this archetypal story in a number of ways. In ancient times, carvers of gems favored the emerald for its rich color and for its combination of durability and ease of carving. Mughal carvers in particular coveted this stone, and the Mughal are known for their exceptional emeralds, which tend to be flat and are generally inscribed with floral patterns or geometric designs. Occasionally, these tablet-shaped gems will bear an inscription, such as a prayer or a holy name.

Ancient lapidaries record other kinds of emeralds bearing engravings and inscriptions too. In Vedic astrology, the emerald is used in fashioning a talisman to Mercury, which grants a variety of favors, including being "the excellent service of scribes and secretaries," thereby linking this stone to writing.[1] There are also stories of emerald tablets, now entombed, that protect against the gaze of serpents.[2]

In more recent times the "emerald cut" is a design chosen to facet stones in order to accentuate their color. While still popular among diamond lovers, it is best reserved for stones of good quality precisely because it emphasizes the color of any stone. The emerald cut is characterized by a deep pavilion and a large, flat facet on the top, which is referred to as a "table" in gemological terminology. The table cut provides a window into which the wearer can gaze and see into the depth of the stone, thereby magnifying the color. This table is symbolically akin to a tablet (derived from the Latin diminutive for *table*), and this cut helps the embodied archetype of the emerald tablet endure even today.

Alchemists believed that the magical inscription on the legendary emerald tablet could be traced back to the beginning of time, while others believed its origin was the time of Atlantis. The text of the *Emerald Tablet* is comprised of roughly fourteen lines, though it varies significantly from one translation to the next. They can be organized a variety of ways and stated in clear or complex language, but the message is unchanged. The author and narrator of the principles on the emerald is a mythical figure named Hermes the Thrice-Great, a master alchemist. The text outlines the major steps of this magnum opus:

The Text on the Tablet

Tis true without lying, certain and most true.

That which is below corresponds to that which is above, and that which is above is like that which is below to accomplish miracles of the One Thing.

And as all things have been and arose from One, through the meditation of One Mind, so all things have their birth from the One through transmutation.

Its father is the Sun, and its mother is the Moon,

The wind carries it in its womb, and the earth is its nurse.

Its power is perfected.

If cast to earth, it will separate earth from fire, the subtle from the gross.

It rises from the earth to the heavens, and returns in descent to the earth thus binding the powers of heaven and earth.

By this work you will acquire the glory of the whole world, and so you will drive away all shadows and blindness.

Its force is above all other forces, for it overcomes every subtle manifestation and penetrates every solid thing.

In this manner, the world was created.

From this come marvelous adaptations of which this is the pattern.

Therefore I am called Hermes Trismegistus, since I have the three
    parts of the wisdom and philosophy of the Universe.

Thus ends the revelation of the work of the Sun.[3]

The opening lines of the *Emerald Tablet* describe what is known
as the "Doctrine of Correspondences," and they serve as the basis for
the esoteric principle "as above, so below." This sets up the remaining
instructions as fitting within their proper orientation in all of creation.
Dennis William Hauck, a widely recognized leader in the field of consciousness studies, writes that

> the relationship . . . here is vertical, and it locates the reader at the
> center of a living interaction between the Above and the Below,
> between heaven and earth. This cosmic axis, the backbone of God,
> is the divine image imprinted on all of creation. It extends infinitely
> upward and infinitely downward, and the only thing clearly defined
> is the center from which the Above and Below stretch outward. It is
> *from this central position* that the powers of Above and Below can be
> observed and put into action.[4]

Emerald as a gemstone relays a similar message to us, if only we can
look in the proper place. The *Emerald Tablet* instructs us to become
centered in the universe, as emerald guides the consciousness into the
center of one's being—the heart. Emerald crystals exhibit a high degree
of symmetry because they belong to the hexagonal crystal class. Their
classic form consists of six elongated prism faces that lay parallel to the
central axis, or c-axis, of the crystal. These six faces meet at equal angles
around the c-axis, and they are united around it.

Emeralds are extremely centering and supportive. The nature of
emeralds had been ascribed to the heart and emotions even before the
New Age adopted color and chakra correspondences for each of the

gemstones used in healing. In today's crystal lore, emerald is one of the premier healers of the heart center, which is the central chakra in our energetic anatomy. In other words, the heart, as the fourth chakra, sits at the midway point along the column of chakras, which extend equally above and below it.

Emerald's hexagonal crystal form echoes traditional associations with the heart center. The heart chakra, known as *Anahata* in Sanskrit, is often depicted as a twelve-petal lotus with a six-pointed star within it. The overall form can be superimposed on emerald's geometry without flaw. Emeralds teach us that the archetype of the emerald tablet first requires the aspiring alchemist to bring full and utter awareness to the heart as the meeting place of above and below, heaven and earth.

This alchemical principle that legend says is engraved on the mythic emerald tablet also tells us that "our everyday lives, as well as those events we perceive as miraculous, are accomplished by the natural interplay of the powers of the Above and Below. In other words, there are no real miracles, only manifestations of the universe's hidden laws."[5] This aligns with the spiritual principle that miracles are the natural order of creation. Only when we can experience a heart-centered point of view can miracles manifest, but the tablet also teaches us that the nature of the heart—that is to say, love—is the driving principle of all actions and reactions in the universe.

One Mind and One Thing

In the lexicon of the text of the *Emerald Tablet,* the terms *One Mind* and *One Thing* have many levels of meaning. On a cursory level, *One Mind* could be defined as God, Creator, Source, et al. On a grander scale, however, *One Mind* can be interpreted as not only Creator, but all of creation, for we all stem from that central source. This mind is not merely a cerebral intellect, as our word *mind* connotes; it is instead a union of heart and mind, just as lapis lazuli co-creates through its archetypes. Rather than being a force of thought and rationality, the One Mind is a truth that can only be known with the heart.

Emerald stresses the heart in all matters. While its green coloration hearkens to ideas of the heart chakra in many modern-day resources, the emerald can be traced back to the heart through its morphology, composition, and historical connections. The chromium to which emerald owes its green color is often associated with physical ailments of the heart and circulatory system, as well as to "encouraging the desire for self-determination," or, more simply: it helps you to put your heart into what you attempt.[6] Surely the universe extended from the One Mind with more than just thought; it must also have been a process encompassing the heart and its capacity to love.

The *One Thing* of the *Emerald Tablet* is a bit more elusive. It is sometimes described as the *prima materia,* or "first matter." This refers to the primordial substance that is undifferentiated, the contents of the void. The One Thing rises, descends, and is made manifest. Emerald's columnar structure identifies the vertical trajectory of the One Thing, and its hexagonal morphology, being the most unified and efficient among crystalline geometries, represents the *prima materia* crystallizing into being.

The remainder of the text of the *Emerald Tablet* serves to illustrate the processes undertaken in the transformation of the One Thing into all that we know. It makes special mention that the driving force of alchemy is above all other forces, and that it drives away shadows and darkness by its light. Surely, this force can only be love in its most primal and unconditional form. Emerald centers our hearts in this divine flow in order to access the same power that is used in the transmutative operation in the alchemical tradition.

Lead into Gold, and Other Miracles

Alchemists of yesteryear are portrayed as seeking the legendary philosopher's stone, a substance that transforms base metal into gold and grants eternal life. The *Emerald Tablet* is generally viewed as the basic text for all works undertaken to create this mythical substance, and the true nature of alchemy can be learned by looking at it through a different lens.

Changing lead into gold is no small feat. Chemists and physicists have mused over the impossibility of such an act, yet the image persists. The true goal of undertaking the magnum opus isn't as simple as becoming wealthy beyond imagination or living indefinitely. Rather, alchemy, like all spiritual arts, helps one engage in a process of self-actualization. Alchemy helps to transform the leaden, base metal of our current state of being into something rarefied and precious, not unlike gold.

Alchemy's goal requires dedication, mindfulness, and plenty of raw material. No mythical alchemist ever managed to create the philosopher's stone in the first try; likewise, it is necessary to apply oneself to personal alchemy time and time again in order to see results—that is why it is called a spiritual practice! Emerald is a powerful catalyst for healing and growth on many levels. It centers the spiritual aspirant in the heart, and it helps one apply the "force above all forces" in every moment of the day.

Decoding the Tablet

Emerald shares many qualities with lapis lazuli in legend and folklore. Emerald was known for soothing the eyes, representing the color of paradise and conferring divine protection from a variety of evils, just like the previous stone in our journey, lapis. Of special importance are those connections that help us decode the tablet in preparation for performing the Great Work of alchemy.

First, many ancient texts ascribe a beneficial influence over the eyes to this green gemstone. It is thought that the Roman emperor Nero watched the gladiators through a lens of pure emerald, ostensibly to improve his vision and soothe his eyes. While it is unlikely that such a large, flawless stone existed, the message runs deeper than merely soothing the eyes. Emerald is a stone for the truth seeker. As such, peering into it magnifies and exposes the inner workings of any endeavor, just as the emerald cut magnifies the color of a gemstone.

The emerald is a lens through which one looks to see the processes underlying form and function. It displays a hexagonal crystal form, and its crystal system is highly ordered. Because hexagons use the least perimeter for a given area, they are found in plentitude in nature. Honeycombs, skin cells, insects' eyes, the scutes of a turtle's shell—all exhibit this hexagonal form, which permits more to be packed into a given space than any other geometric form. Because of this, the emerald, whose crystal system is so precise, offers a glimpse into what is hidden behind the surface.

Emeralds are luminous stones; they are often connected to truth and justice, as well as to divine order. Their crystal form permits secrets to be revealed because it holds another geometric key: when exposed to X-ray diffraction, the morphology of beryl crystals such as emeralds reveal the Flower of Life.[7] The Flower of Life represents the first informational system of creation; it is a geometric rendering of All That Is and can be said to represent the nature of space and time.

Connecting to the emerald as in the alchemical text the *Emerald Tablet* is not merely about following complex, symbolic instructions for creating the philosopher's stone. Emerald reveals the interconnectedness of all life through the one force that is greater than all others. Like the joined circles in the Flower of Life, emerald teaches that all of creation is similarly interdependent and linked to the power of the heart. Truly, the whole of alchemy can be reduced to listening to the heart, to love, and this is a truth so simple that it could be written on an emerald of any size.

MEDITATION
REFLECTING ON THE TABLET

Choose an emerald with a flat plane before commencing this exercise. It can be perfectly smooth or not; it does not have to be perfectly flat, the choice is yours. I have a polished, opaque emerald that I use for this exercise, an oversized, emerald-cut stone. If you have a specific area of life that needs some clarity or guidance, you may focus on that at the appropriate moment.

Hold the stone cradled in both hands and gaze at its surface. As you stare with unfocused eyes, imagine that any surface etchings or inclusions within the stone are sacred writings in some unknown language. Gently allow your eyes to close and stroke the stone with your thumb or forefinger, as if reading Braille. Imagine that the words light up and travel along your finger, up your arm, and are deposited in your heart center.

In your heart, a secret is revealed to you as this process continues; you see the perfection and connectedness of all life. Continue to fill your heart with this emerald green luminescence and ask your emerald tablet to help you solve whatever personal challenge or opportunity you may be facing. This guidance may come in the form of a symbolic answer, or perhaps you will see or hear the words in answer to your question.

Thank your emerald for its alchemical guidance. When you are satisfied, hold the stone to your heart, inhale deeply, and exhale the emerald light into the world around you. Return your awareness to the room and open your eyes.

EMERALD AS AN ARCHETYPE: THE GRAIL STONE

The Holy Grail persists in myth and legend because it represents the mystery of resurrection and magic. In modern times the grail has permeated pop culture through the fictional character of Indiana Jones, the movie *The Da Vinci Code,* and the British surreal comedy group Monty Python. In most tales, the grail itself is a sacred cup or chalice from the Last Supper. This same grail was said to catch some of the blood of Christ during his crucifixion, and it was passed on from one generation to the next for safekeeping. The grail changes form over the ages; sometimes it is a plate or dish, while at other times it is a goblet. Sometimes simple, sometimes radiantly ornate, the Holy Grail is frequently associated with gemstones, particularly the emerald.

The most prolific retelling of the grail mythos is by Wolfram von Eschenbach, who built on the earlier stories of Chretien de Troyes and Robert de Boron in his description of the sacred vessel. In Eschenbach's epic poem *Parzival,* the grail takes the form of a dish or plate carved from green stone. The grail story combines elements of Christian symbolism with Celtic mythology, and it is encoded with symbols and messages that evoke the nature of the archetype of emerald.

The Holy Grail is purported to have restorative powers. Anyone who drinks from this chalice will have life everlasting. It can heal any illness and stave off death itself. It is considered linked to the phoenix, "the fabled stone by whose power the Phoenix of classical mythology rises in rebirth from its ashes."[8] It is also written that the "Grail provides sustenance, food, and drink" as well as salvation itself.[9] For some scholars, the grail is a metaphor for Christ.

Legend has it that this holy gem once adorned the brow of the personification of the morning star. Lucifer, once the most beautiful and loyal of the host of angels in heaven, owned this emerald crystal and wore it in a diadem or crown. This angel's name comes from the Latin *Vulgate,* meaning "Light-bearer"; it was *Phosphoros,* or "Light-carrier" in Greek before that. Lucifer was especially radiant, as was his fabled and precious treasure. In the Judeo-Christian tradition it is said that in the rebellion that ensued, after which Lucifer was cast out of heaven, his crown was broken, "and the Great Emerald was loosened and fell like a green meteor in a shower of light to earth."[10] It was this gleaming gem that eventually made its way to the Last Supper. Its noble provenance is said to have included the Queen of Sheba, who first claimed it from where it fell. The queen purportedly later gave this stone to King Solomon. The trail of Lucifer's gem ultimately leads to Christ, for the *lapis exillis* would eventually be fashioned into the Holy Grail, and it would figure prominently into a great act of transfiguration.

The grail itself serves as a sacred crucible in which the work of the alchemist may take place. Into it one must place the *prima materia* for the Great Work. The sacred chalice symbolizes the cauldron of transformation that the alchemist must use to achieve liberation through transmutation. Out of the Great Work is born the philosopher's stone, and the sacred elixir of life can be distilled.

The work of alchemy parallels the grail legend in a number of ways. First, the Holy Grail is said to endow anyone who drinks from it with life everlasting. It also spreads joy, cures all illnesses, and serves as a vehicle for rebirth on all levels. It has long been equated with the phoenix, whose qualities of being reborn to achieve immortality are found in this cup. "The Grail, then, is the gemstone of all gemstones; it is the stone that makes death, in pre-Christian 'heathen' terms, into a molting of feathers. With new feathers, the soul flies again."[11] Just like the Holy Grail, the secret art of alchemy is said to elicit immortality, cure disease, and transform base substances into their higher forms. Emerald serves to unite these two archetypes through its resonance with healing and rejuvenating body, mind, and spirit.

As the cup used in the Last Supper, the grail is said to have contained the blood of Christ. As Jesus held aloft a vessel of wine and decreed it to be his blood, the sacrament of Communion was initiated. This continues in liturgical traditions today, wherein bread and wine are transfigured into the body and blood of the Christ. In Catholic teachings, this is the basis of the doctrine of transubstantiation, in which the Eucharist and sacramental wine are not merely symbols but are transformed (transubstantiated) into the actual body and blood of the Savior. This act of transubstantiation is considered a divine mystery in other Christian denominations; it is an act of alchemy that seeks to refine the wine and bread into the Christ. The grail symbolically serves as the vessel for the host; it is the vehicle on which the transformation occurs. Similarly, emerald works to transform our own hearts and bodies such that we can achieve a perfected state. Through an act of divine mystery, the love that flows throughout the universe converges within the human heart and refines the totality of the human being.

The Grail as an Altar

Some scholars posit that the grail known to Wolfram von Eschenbach was not an actual cup; rather, it was a dish or plate that held the Eucharist during liturgical rites. Descriptions of the Holy Grail as a stone indicate that it was portable, engraved with writing or images, and was an actual object rather than an abstraction or ideal. It was said to make known the will of God by means of the writing that appears on it.[12] This description lends itself to the probability that the grail stone may actually have been, at least in some stories, a portable altar, known as a *lapis itinerarii*.[13] These altars, whose name translates as "stone for travel/journey," were usually consecrated with a piece of the Eucharist that was sealed within them. In this manner, even the grail as an altar stone would have held the body and blood of Christ. Because they could be used in processionals or on long journeys, the *lapides itinerarii* could serve as the focal point for ritual outside the walls of a church.

Emerald, too, shows the way to connecting to the divine mystery without being enclosed by a man-made structure. Emerald, as a stone that is intimately connected to the heart, helps to reconnect the heart to the natural order, which exists as an expression of divine love. In this way, emerald reminds the heart to empty itself of any frequency that is not in resonance with this state, thereby allowing it to become the proverbial empty vessel.

As one works with emerald and its teachings, it helps to awaken the heart to the luminous nature of love and its ability to transmute unconditionally. Emerald serves to activate the heart as the Holy Grail. In legend and lore, knights and nobles sought the grail far and wide, but the only place to look for the archetypal grail is within. This transforms the gross nature of the human heart into a refined state; it then becomes the altar that receives the host. Our hearts, as empty chalices, become vessels for being filled with the nature of the Christ. This internal alchemy permits the human being to receive the love of all that is, and Creator fills and sanctifies our hearts through the mystery of emeralds.

Truly, emerald shows that with love, all things are possible. It rarefies and refines the nature of our body, mind, and spirit to endow us with the qualities of immortality. This does not mean that the goal of alchemy is to live without dying; instead, emerald shows that through the experience of unconditional love and compassion we meet and know the nature of eternity on an intimate, heartfelt level.

MEDITATION

THE GRAIL OF THE HEART

Sit in a comfortable position with your emerald of choice. Begin the meditation with a few relaxed breaths before picking up the stone. As you enter a more relaxed state, gently hold the emerald in your receptive hand (typically the nondominant hand), and gradually move it toward your heart center. When it makes contact with your chest, hold the stone in place with both hands, one on top of the other. Imagine that as you breathe in, the green light of the emerald penetrates your chest and begins to illuminate your heart.

With each breath, the heart is brighter and brighter. Each time you exhale, release any thought or sensation that arises that is in conflict with peace and compassion. Simply allow the emerald to empty your heart of disharmonious energies. When the process feels as though it has reached its peak, hold the image for a few moments as you breathe in the emerald light.

Next, direct your attention to the heavens above; imagine that you can see the unconditional love, support, and compassion of Creator raining down everywhere. You can visualize this in any way that feels right to you. Allow it to enter through the crown of your head and flow downward into the vessel of your heart. Each breath in fills your heart center with more love and compassion than it has ever known. Allow it to overflow and fill your entire being. As it reaches full capacity, allow any additional love to flow through you and into the earth beneath you. Breathe in and out like this, with each in-breath allowing more and more love to flow into you and the earth. When you feel ready to draw the meditation to a close, exhale all the green light back into the emerald.

As the green light fades away, your entire being shines with golden light. Breathe deeply and return your awareness to the room.

Although this is a simple visualization, the effects can be profound. As the emerald ray fills your heart, it initiates the process of alchemy. With regular practice this technique can refine your entire being and fashion you into the perfect vessel for transformation and transmutation.

EMERALD AS AN ARCHETYPE: ENTERING EDEN

In the traditions of medieval lapidaries, emeralds owe their origin to fantastic places. Sometimes they are sourced from the nests of gryphons; at other times they came to our world through the waters of the Phison River, one of the four bodies of water that are said to have flowed through the Garden of Eden. This connection to Eden follows emerald throughout its history, and it furnishes our journey with a final archetype to contemplate.

Eden, as the archetypal and prototypical paradise from which humankind is descended, was a lush and peaceful region. It is here that the first humans incarnated and where the emerald ultimately seeks to take us on our journey. The Garden of Eden is the birthplace of not only humanity and the rest of life, it also serves as the locus of the Fall, and the church's doctrine of original sin subsequently arose out of this. Worldwide, the origin stories of the emerald are no stranger to Edenic lands, from the biblical account of Creation to the myths of the peoples of Central and South America.

The native people of Colombia, the Muzo, have several myths surrounding the emerald. Among them are stories of the first woman and man, named Fura and Tena, respectively. When they broke the commandment given to them by Creator, they suffered a gruesome fate. After Tena's death, Fura's tears crystallized into mountains of emerald. The Creator took pity on them and restored their lives, granting safe passage to the paradise among the emerald mountains.[14]

The Islamic scriptures also imagine a paradise of emeralds. In fact, it is said that their vision of paradise is "carpeted with emeralds."[15] Similarly, emeralds are believed to make up the pebbles in the rivers of paradise, and Mohammed's vision of heaven includes a tree that bears fruit and leaves of precious emerald gems.[16] Similarly, biblical lore suggests that emeralds also line the bed of the river Phison.

Throughout lapidary history, emerald gemstones have lent themselves to being engraved with foliate and floral patterns. The verdant glow of emerald evokes images of nature that would entice jewelers to sculpt flowers, leaves, grapes, and animals out of gem-quality crystals. The connection to a paradisical plot of nature, one without greed, death, illness, or discontent, aligns itself with the message and history of emerald.

The Fall of Humanity

When Adam and Eve ate of the fruit of the Tree of Knowledge of Good and Evil, they were cast from Eden. Death, disease, and pain were all brought into the world. The tradition of oppression and devaluation of all things feminine can be traced to episodes just like this one. Truly, the biblical event known as the Fall was much more internal, rather than a literal moment of weakness due to a crafty snake.

The Fall was begotten when separation entered human consciousness. The Tree of Knowledge of Good and Evil is a representation of dichotomy and segregation: good from evil, light from dark, God from human being. The parable of Eden represents the fall of consciousness, wherein humankind lost sight of its collective divinity and started to view the divine as outside our being. Emerald shadows this message with its own fall from paradise to the earth.

When the light-bearer, Lucifer of the morning star, was cast from heaven, Archangel Michael struck his crown, thus sending the gemstone it held to the earthly realms. When the angelic adversary is cast out, it represents the conflict humans experience with their own divinity. The ego is the adversary; because of its rebelliousness, our inner spark of divinity is apparently stripped from us as we experience a consciousness that perceives the illusion of separation as truth.

The symbol of the morning star is especially relevant to a thorough understanding of the symbolism at work in this artfully encoded vignette. "Morning star" is the epithet for the planet Venus, as it is often seen gleaming like a star during the dawn's golden light. In the mystery traditions such as are found in Theosophy, Venus is regarded as being home to the group of beings known as the Kumaras. The Kumaras are angels, sages, and teachers; to the Hindus they were often depicted as Nagaraja, or "king snake,"[17] which clearly lays the foundation for the biblical story of the serpent. In Japan the story is retold as the embodiment of the earth, called Mao-son, comes to its home within a mountain known as Kurama, from the planet Venus.

The fall of the emerald also "signifies the fall of the planetary Logos, which moves from Venus to the Earth—representing an enormous sacrifice and a true descent into the abysses of our world."[18] The planetary Logos is essentially the original law or blueprint governing the makeup and mission of our planet. The Logos descended from its place in the heavens, on its throne on the morning star, and came to the physical plane of our dense planet. It can be said that "Lucifer's lost emerald presages the loss of Eden by Adam and Eve" as well as being a roadmap for restoring the state of consciousness prior to the Fall.[19]

Rebirthing the Goddess

Venus is a primal goddess archetype, preserved in Greek and Roman mythology as a goddess of love and romance. The planet shares its name with her, and the astrological qualities of Venus are femininity and love. The role of Venus is greater than simply being the bright sign of the light-bearer or the homeland of the Logos of Earth. The goddess archetype runs throughout the myths of emerald's creation and properties, and working with emerald helps to heal the divine feminine, thus restoring it to its rightful place along the journey to paradise.

In the grail myths, women play an important role. For example, in

Eschenbach's *Parzival,* only women are shown carrying the grail stone. "Wolfram assigns to women a major role . . . In his story, women are not equal to men—they are ahead of men. In the quest . . . to become real human beings, they show the way."[20] The influence of the feminine principle extends even to the grail itself. The grail, as a chalice or cup, is a motif repeated in cultures around the world to represent the archetypal goddess. In Neopagan rites, altars are typically adorned with a chalice or goblet as a representation of the Mother Goddess. In Tantric Buddhism, the bell, an upside-down cup, signifies the feminine or dakini principle, which is counterposed with the dorje, the guru or wand, a masculine principle.

The emerald has known many goddesses throughout time. In South America, the native Peruvians knew the Mother Goddess as Umiña; her image was a gigantic crystal of emerald, the size of an ostrich egg.[21] Her priests were documented as gathering smaller emeralds, seen as her children, which were given to this idol as offerings. In Egypt, Isis reputedly wore an emerald in her headband.[22] Overall, emeralds and other green gemstones "have been invested with mystic connotations, possibly because of their widely recognized association with the Mother Goddess in antiquity," and this connection to the divine feminine serves to offer healing to those who walk the spiritual path.[23]

One author writes that the emerald "is one of the most feminine representatives of the mineral kingdom: the Shakti, the divine mother, and the goddess."[24] Emerald serves to restore the mysteries of the divine feminine to their original role; just as the Holy Grail resurrects all who drink from it, the chalice can help rebirth the Great Goddess within the human psyche. The chalice, or grail, is the very womb in which our soul is incubated. The Divine Mother is often appointed the role of Mother Earth, for all we see and know is born from her.

Emerald reminds us that when the planetary Logos fell from Venus, a rift between male and female was first forged. Furthermore, when in the Fall Adam and Eve were cast out of paradise, the divine nature of humanity was forgotten. Emerald can gradually undo the damage inherited from the Fall by revealing and restoring the Goddess to her throne. Only by offering respect, love, and support to all genders can the Goddess be honored as equally as the masculine principle of God the Father. Emerald, long associated with truth and with justice, helps to balance the scales both personally and socially.

Childlike Innocence

Before the Fall, the natural state was one of innocence and freedom. There was no fear, no pain, and no unhappiness. Emerald shows that the natural state to which we can aspire is identical to the Edenic condition. The most regal of green stones can be viewed as the supreme gem of resurrection. It helps to heal and restore the heart to its initial state of innocence, all the while helping to raise the consciousness of its user.

Emerald is best known for healing the emotional field and for balancing the heart center. Alchemically, the *Emerald Tablet* guides the process of rarefaction by welcoming our tarnished and oxidized selves of base metal into the crucible of the Great Work. Therein, we are transmuted to the golden state of innocence through the virtue of unconditional love. In the mode of joy and compassion that accompanies this transformation, we experience a total lack of judgment, partisanship, and bias.

The evolution of the psyche yearns for the maternal influence of goddess energy, and emerald will usher this to us for healing and wholeness. As we embrace the wholeness of the divine, with masculine and feminine as equal parts of the cosmic unity, separation consciousness and duality fall by the wayside. Through the alchemical modus operandi, the human heart is restored to completeness and integrity. Our hearts literally fill with the outpouring of divine love. This presence is most felt when the grail helps us to empty ourselves of any attachment that could keep us out of the metaphorical state of Eden. "The spiritual Grail may be thought of as the awakened and fully realized intelligence of the human heart," and in its fully awakened state our consciousness returns to being heart-centered rather than head-centered.[25]

In the story of the prototypical emerald in the crown of Lucifer, the emerald was located above the seat of the mind. At the time of Lucifer's fall from heaven, the emerald fell from his crown; this represents the rendering of the mind as the highest perceived function of humankind. Even the descent from Venus draws a close parallel: if Venusian energies connect to the heart center and the emotional body, leaving them behind signifies an emphasis on the gross, material plane and supports the primacy of the mind over the heart.

Emerald's archetypes are the tools for applying the lessons taught by the previous stones. They help us to cope with the real-world relevance of these teachings. The *Emerald Tablet* is our map, the set of instructions for finding the path. The Holy Grail is our vehicle; it is the vessel in which the journey of transformation of the human heart is undertaken. Finally, Eden is our destination. Like any spiritual discipline, Eden serves as the setting for the whole journey rather than merely its final haven.

MEDITATION

FINDING EDEN

Select any emerald that you like, natural or polished. Find a comfortable place to sit undisturbed and close your eyes while holding the stone. In your mind's eye, picture the emerald growing larger. As it grows, it becomes more transparent, appearing to be lit from within. Continue to picture the emerald expanding in size until it is at least the size of a house.

On the side of the crystal, you see a doorway or gate. Approach this entrance to the stone and ask it to share its mysteries with you. The door opens, and you feel a magnetic pull toward the interior of the stone. Once inside, you see a lush garden; each and every inclusion in the stone appears to be a living plant or creature. Take in the scene with each of your senses. What does it look like? How does it feel to your hands and feet? What is the aroma? What sounds or music do you hear? If you feel adventurous, taste one of the plants, knowing that everything here is safe.

At your feet there is path, indicated by mossy green stepping stones. Follow them into the heart of the garden. You come across a secluded area ringed by tall, flowering bushes. Walk around this circle of plants until an opening appears. Bow your head as you enter, and you are greeted by the emerald goddess. She offers you a token of gratitude for visiting her and sharing her goddess energy with the world.

You may ask of her any question you have or approach her for healing. She surrounds you with a warm, emerald-colored light, which dissolves all your troubles and leaves you gleaming with innocence. When you have finished, thank the goddess, retrace your steps, and return your awareness to your physical body. Allow the emerald to return to its normal size. Take a few gentle breaths and open your eyes.

THE EMERALD IN CRYSTAL HEALING

Emerald's long tradition of therapeutic uses tends to focus on two main avenues: physical healing and emotional well-being. The knowledge of its curative powers dates back to the earliest emerald discoveries in ancient Egypt, and with the proliferation of this gemstone throughout the world its medicinal properties also spread.

On the physical level, specimens of emerald have been used to soothe the eyes, to rejuvenate the body, and to offer healing through its connection to the natural world. Emerald's rich, leafy color has been noted for providing a source of healing energy. In the methodology of gemstone therapy, in which only refined stones meeting specific parameters for quality are used, emerald is the stone par excellence for physical healing. It reportedly "brings life, nourishment, and healing" on a corporeal level.[26]

Emerald works through the third ray, the green ray, according to traditions of Western occultism. According to the system of seven rays described by Alice Bailey, the third ray, which is ruled by Saturn,* is the

---

*Gemstones are frequently given multiple astrological correspondences, as they are multidimensional tools. Emerald displays a Venusian energy in light of its heart-centered, loving influence. It can also be relegated to Saturn's rule because its verdant color represents the greenery of Earth, and, therefore, the world of physical form. Saturn represents structure, form, and the crystallization of ideas. In Ayurveda, this green gem is associated with Mercury, instead, as a result of its clarity and brilliance, which represent the Mercurial strengths of intellect and clear communication. In this manner, emerald is able to embody multiple planetary archetypes.

ray of intellect. Emerald, its chief stone, therefore helps to remediate the manner in which one thinks. It bestows clarity to the mind, broadens one's perspective, and alleviates feelings of mental fogginess. Ultimately, this clarity and understanding trickles down to feelings of connection with the world around you. The gardenlike inclusions found within emerald crystals create a sympathetic resonance with nature. Because of this, wearing or meditating with emeralds awakens the threads that connect one to all of life. The green ray, as taught in gemstone therapy, provides nourishment and regeneration to all living things. It works first by targeting the areas of greatest disharmony in the body, where it "neutralizes and disintegrates the disharmony that manifests as disease and discomfort."[27]

Traditional sources also record the use of emerald in healing the heart, alleviating strain on the eyes, and for promoting the healthy functioning of the sexual organs. The gentle, candescent gleam of polished emerald is truly soothing to gaze at, and ancient writers attributed emerald's healing powers to this beauty.

Working with lower-quality emeralds such as those commonly available in raw and tumbled forms can help to anchor the user more fully in the body. They are denser and less transparent than their gem-grade siblings, and the healing nature of these stones is necessarily less intense. These emeralds are well-suited to applications of grounding, centering, and strengthening the physical level of one's being.

Emeralds in history are famed for their impact on the heart and the emotions. Medieval lapidary texts regard the famed green gem as ensuring marital fidelity, promoting love, and granting peace and virtue. Emeralds are known for having a transformational effect on all levels of the heart and mind. The vivid green hue nourishes and soothes the inner makeup of anyone who wears emerald. Emeralds work to heal the heart center by overriding the seed thoughts that are responsible for unhappiness, despondency, and disconnectedness. These can manifest emotionally as depression, feelings of isolation, and helplessness. Physically, they can manifest as illness and injury.

The longer one works with emerald, the deeper its energies can penetrate to the level at which the cause of the problem exists; gradually, this gem unravels the emotional patterns that root themselves in our psyches and beget sickness.

One of emerald's greatest gifts revolves around forgiveness and atonement. While lapis helps to return the soul of humankind to its rightful place on the throne in the heavens, emerald helps heal the accessory damage incurred during the Fall. Through atonement, it is possible to cultivate inner grace and benevolence. A conscious practice of gratitude permits one to share the gift of grace outward, creating ripples in the sea of human hearts seeking wholeness on our planet. Through the function of atonement, emerald heals shame and resentment. It aspires to transmute these base emotions into higher expressions such as gratitude, pride, and respect. The alchemical nature of this crystalline ally prevails over the base elements through acts of virtue. Wolfram's *Parzival* equates the nature of the Holy Grail to a baptismal font, and many traditions about emerald also contain a similar, aqueous theme. Emerald washes away our faults and those of our karmic and familial bonds in order to permit us to fulfill our mission with a pure and resplendent heart.

Emerald is a multifaceted healing stone. Though it has been prized for creating the benefits of good health and physical vitality, it activates the intelligence of the heart too. Connecting deeply to emerald's archetypes opens the heart and raises the consciousness to a point wherein the intellect and emotional field are in perfect harmony. Emerald is an ally for anyone who can benefit from an understanding of the sentiments underlying any situation or opportunity. Emerald can help to perfect the unified field of the heart and mind, and offers a fair and just perspective on any topic.

Emerald is often touted as being a stone that represents truth and justice. It brings peace to the mind and joy to the heart. Emerald's essence opens the doorway to authenticity and sincerity; it helps you to be true to your own heart and true to your mission on the earth.

Likewise, emerald is the perfect vessel for exploring your sense of purpose and alchemically aligning it with the Higher Power.

Varieties of Emerald

African Emerald

African emeralds span the entire history of the gemstone. The earliest known emeralds came from the lost mines of Cleopatra, situated in Jabal Sukayt and Jabal Zabārah, near the Red Sea coast east of Aswān. These mines have subsequently been found. Nowadays, several African nations supply a large amount of the gem trade's emeralds. Many of the stones currently available from Africa tend to have a bluer color than those from Colombia.

African emeralds are often richer in iron; as such they are more emboldening and corporeally oriented. Iron, ruled by Mars, is the complement to the Venusian quality for which emeralds are known. Because of this, these stones can promote a better dynamic and smoother communication between couples. These green gems are also rooted firmly in tradition, and connecting to their energy can instill respect for customs and for one's heritage. Some have theorized that Africa may have been the location of the Garden of Eden, and these stones connect most closely to the archetype of Eden.

Brazilian Emerald

Brazilian emeralds can be found in a variety of greens. Many good-quality green beryls are mined in Brazil, but only those with chromium or vanadium are considered to be true emeralds by most in the gem trade. Given that Brazil is the original source for vanadium-bearing stones, we will address only those, and how they differ from other emeralds. It may be necessary to have some emeralds tested to determine the exact source of their coloration.

Brazilian emerald confers the same overall qualities as those from other locations. In addition to representing the archetypes of emerald mentioned in this chapter, vanadium provides specific relief from inflammation and irritation of skin, eyes, and respiratory organs.[28] Held over an afflicted area, this gem can relieve the buildup of fluid and toxins experienced during inflammation and congestion. Due to its vanadium content, Brazilian emerald is also useful for loosening the hold of unnecessary restraint. It can loosen the bonds of unhealthy social ties, for example, in unhealthy relationships or from being overly concerned by social obligations. Additionally, while all emeralds are effective at physical healing, this particular stone galvanizes the rejuvenation and revitalization of the body at a cellular level, restoring youthfulness and vitality while simultaneously eliminating disease.

Cat's Eye Emerald

Cat's eye emeralds are unusual and uncommon members of the beryl group. They are characterized by thin, fibrous inclusions or transparent growth tubules growing parallel to one another, which reveal a chatoyant, or cat's eye effect, upon polishing. The raw crystal form is often striated and terminates with a pyramidal apex. Under very rare circumstances, trapiche emeralds (see below) can also exhibit the same chatoyancy when polished.

Cat's eyes are stones with interesting optical phenomena; the fibrous structures within their crystalline matrix conduct light much like fiber-optic cables. They often have a soft, velvety sheen that appears to be lit from within. The cat's eye emerald is a visionary stone; it helps one to dream bigger than ever and promotes innovation, intuition, and insight. Working with it creates a clear path for seeing with the heart and for bringing forth tenderness and discernment in spiritual pursuits.

Trapiche Emerald

Hailing from Colombia, the trapiche emerald contains carbon-based inclusions radiating from the center of the stone in six rays, often stemming around a central ring. The name of this stone comes from the Spanish word indicating a type of wheel used to grind cane in the production of sugar, as the inclusions in these emeralds closely resemble a wheel.

Trapiche emeralds are lovely stones that create harmony and focus. The radiating spokes can be viewed as moving inward, toward a common goal at the heart of any circumstance, or outward, into the world of form. The stone helps the separate pieces of any situation or organization come together and work in unison, like the cogs in a machine. The hexagonal symmetry, green color, and heart or core outlined by carbon connect the emerald to the heart center. Trapiche emeralds are useful in correcting blockages or misalignments of the heart chakra, and this can result in healthier relationships. Trapiches encourage us to put our heart into any effort in order to enjoy a happier, more fruitful result. Working with this variety of emerald can help you find sweetness and contentment in the everyday workings of life.

Related Stones

Aquamarine

Aquamarine is a blue to green sister beryl of emerald. The characteristic color spectrum is derived from iron, which along with chromium or vanadium is found in many emeralds. Greener gems are often heated to lighten their color and render them more blue, but very green examples of aquamarine can be an excellent substitute for emerald.

Aquamarine emphasizes the qualities of water, after which it takes its name. It helps to cleanse, release and purify on all levels. Aquamarine can help the mind release its hold on old, outmoded beliefs in order to gain a clearer perspective and achieve a state of illumination and inspiration. Aquamarine helps you stay centered in the flow of universal abundance, and it engenders trust in this state through a truthful perspective on the ebb and flow of all things.

Physically, aquamarine is very detoxifying. Not only does it relate to the flowing properties of water, it actually helps you return to a state of "energetic liquidity."[29] Aquamarine is a versatile tool, and it has a refreshing effect on all levels of existence. Partnered with emerald, it can foster presence of mind, emotional balance, and deep healing at the physical level.

Demantoid Garnet

Sometimes called "Uralian emerald" in the gemstone industry (after the Ural Mountains in Russia, where this gemstone is found), this member of the garnet clan derives its color from chromium. The demantoid is a variety of andradite garnet, which is rich in calcium and iron. Its name is derived from diamond, referring to its brilliance and high refractive index. True demantoids are rare, and they often contain horsetail inclusions as indications of their veracity.

Demantoid garnets are perhaps the brightest green gemstones available. They are a rich emerald green due to a mixture of chromium and iron. Overall, garnets are generally grounding and supportive of our physical bodies. Green demantoids serve to anchor the green ray in the physical body; the cubic crystal structure and high specific gravity of demantoid garnets serve as a means of grounding and stabilizing the influence of this energy into physical reality, thus enabling the positive influence of the green ray to manifest more concretely. They are nourishing and refreshing. Considered to resonate with a more masculine energy than emerald, demantoid garnets offer balance when used in conjunction with their beryl counterparts. They are highly energetic and are observed to have a fiery quality that "generates at an atomically high-powered rate of oscillation."[30] Its high level of energy, as well as the absolutist nature of its cubic crystal system, can make this gemstone a formidable teacher. It is said to "lovingly, persistently inform us that life is growth and stagnation is death," and as a result it is a stone that promotes not only growth but also maturity.[31] It can offer a turning point in one's growth, and it helps crystallize one's goals into tangible outcomes.

Dioptase

Occasionally referred to as "copper emerald," this uncommon stone radiates an energy comparable to that of the emerald. In natural light it is a true emerald green, but in artificial light dioptase displays a markedly teal color. It is generally too soft to cut, and large crystals are not common. Nonetheless, this mineral offers bountiful support in its natural form.

Dioptase, a complex silicate that contains copper, supports the mission of emerald by bringing its energy directly into the heart center. Copper is astrologically related to Venus, a planet often equated with the emerald. It is a vibrant, heart-illuminating stone, one I always associate with forgiveness. Dioptase can help to locate parts of our auras that are torn as a result of emotional trauma, as well as areas with accumulations of toxic thoughts or feelings, and it helps to gently repair them. It is soft, feminine, and loving in all of its actions.

Moldavite

Moldavite, briefly mentioned in chapter 1, is a naturally occurring glass that resulted from the impact of a meteorite. This gorgeous green gem is typically found in beautifully etched forms in the Czech Republic. This naturally occurring etching is likely erosion as a result of soil chemistry. These etchings may also superficially resemble writing, such as that found on the legendary *Emerald Tablet*. While academics do not agree on the exact nature of moldavite's formation, it is likely that moldavite rained down in its current location after the meteoric impact that first created it. For this reason, it shares a special link to the Holy Grail, an emerald-colored stone that fell to Earth.

Moldavite shares many characteristics with the archetypes of emerald. It may well have been the prototype for the myth of the emerald in Lucifer's crown, which later became the Holy Grail. Because some versions of the *Emerald Tablet* text describe the legendary emerald tablet as having been poured into a mold while molten, these retellings also insinuate that the tablet was fashioned of green glass rather than a true emerald. Moldavite fits the description for both of these archetypes.

Moldavite is often described among crystal enthusiasts as a high-vibration stone, one that even the least sensitive of persons can feel. It has an energy that is characteristic of many of the other high-vibe stones: ungrounded, elevating, transformational, and strongly spiritual. The effects of working with moldavite generally include enhanced psychic perception, more vivid or lucid dreams, greater activity of the higher chakras, enhanced spiritual growth, and increased ability to communicate with nonphysical beings. Many have attested to the presence of an extraterrestrial consciousness or intelligence that can be accessed through this gemstone.

Structurally speaking, moldavite is a stone for accessing the power of the void. The womblike nature of the void perfectly fits into the archetype of the Holy Grail, whose nature as a chalice easily represents the womb of the Mother Goddess. Moldavite helps in the rebirth of higher consciousness through the destructive and reconstructive nature of the void itself. It awakens the heart as the vessel for actualizing the initial spark of alchemy; by doing so it initiates change and transformations from the inside out.

Moldavite is truly a transformational stone. It can be used to connect the archetypes of the emerald to those of obsidian. As such, it lends power, courage, and decisiveness to emerald when they are paired. Begin connecting to emerald first, then try introducing the energy of this star-born stone to magnify the effects of your work.

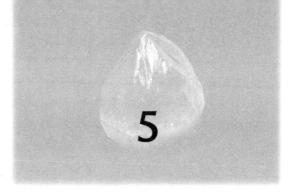

5

AMETHYST

Temperance and Alchemy

Violet and purple gems are appreciably rare when compared to the multitude of other colors available from mines around the world. In light of this, amethyst, a violet member of the quartz family, has virtually always been in fashion. At one point the value of fine amethyst rivaled that of diamonds; royalty, noblemen, and heads of state esteemed this violet stone because of its royal color.

Chemically speaking, amethyst is an impure variety of one of nature's most abundant minerals, quartz. This oxide of silica is the basic unit of most silicate bases found in a multitude of combinations forming many related minerals. Quartz is durable, plentiful, and found worldwide. Trace impurities and inclusions of other minerals account for a wide variety of colors, diaphaneity, and morphology. Quartz forms as euhedral crystals, microcrystalline and cryptocrystalline masses, druses (incrustations of small crystals on the surface of a rock or mineral), nodules, and grains in many rocks.

Amethyst derives its color primarily from iron, as well as from its unique growth structure. Originally, scientists believed that the source of amethyst's color was manganese, although no amount of testing could yield any trace of the element in its lattice. While there is some general agreement on iron being the source of the violet color, the same element is responsible for a number of other shades in quartz, such as the golden, yellowy brown and orange colors of citrine. The exact nature of amethyst's color centers, and the effect of other trace elements, has not yet been entirely worked out by science.[1]

Most forms of amethyst, as well as other iron-tinged quartz, are subject to a special type of twinned growth. Optically speaking, all quartz typically forms as either right- or left-handed. What this means is that the direction of growth of the crystal lattice is either clockwise or counterclockwise. Generally speaking, a given specimen of quartz is oriented in a single direction; amethyst and similar quartzes, however, are exceptions to this rule. Because ions of iron are too large to fit into the basic unit of quartz's crystal lattice, the crystal reconciles the presence of iron by switching back and forth between left-handed and right-handed lattices in a pattern called Airy's spiral, named for its discoverer Sir George Biddell Airy, an English astronomer. Where the two opposing directions meet as distinct layers, there exists just enough room for the iron to squeeze in. This results in unique optical patterns that are mostly visible when thin cross-sections are viewed under polarized light. It may be possible that these phenomena also contribute to the distinctive color of amethyst.

Amethyst is found in a variety of locations worldwide: Ontario, Canada (Thunder Bay is the largest amethyst mine in North America); Mexico; Brazil; Bolivia; France; South Africa; Russia; India; Kenya; and Japan. In the United States amethyst can be found in the Mazatzal Mountain region in Arizona; southwest New Mexico; Red Feather Lakes, near Ft. Collins, Colorado; Amethyst Mountain, Texas; Yellowstone National Park; Delaware County, Pennsylvania; Haywood County, North Carolina; Deer Hill and Stow, Maine; and in the Lake Superior regions of Minnesota, Wisconsin, and Michigan. Most localities produce distinctive growth habits that serve as indicators of their provenance. The morphology of many amethysts, especially those from Canada, Uruguay, and much of Brazil, lack the long prism faces that run parallel to the central axis within the crystal form. Instead, they are clustered together so closely that only the facets of the termination are well formed. Amethysts from many other locations may have elongated c-axes.

Traditionally, this violet quartz has been held in high regard for its striking color and for being eminently carvable. Ancient amethyst cylinder seals, drinking vessels, intaglios, and engraved amulets attest to the perennial popularity and high esteem placed on this regal gem. Amethyst has often been associated with the spiritual side of life, for its color is reminiscent of both royalty and arcane, esoteric teachings. For this reason it has been used as a charm against witchcraft and enchantments, for protecting the virtues of holy men and women, and for parting the veil between ordinary consciousness and the realm of the gods.

AMETHYST AS AN ARCHETYPE:
TEMPERANCE

Amethyst's name is derived from Greek, *a methustos,* meaning "not drunken." The etymology of the word can be traced back to an episode in Greek mythology featuring a nymph named Ametis and her pursuant, the god of wine, Dionysus. The myth begins as Dionysus makes an unreciprocated advance toward the nymph, who is en route to perform adorations at the temple of Artemis. After being rejected, the god began to chase Ametis, and some versions of the story include pursuit with hounds. Ametis, in sheer terror, cries out to the goddess Artemis for intervention. The goddess takes pity on her faithful supplicant and transforms the nymph into white quartz to prevent her from befalling any harm. In a rage that he cannot have the object of his desire, Dionysus throws his token cup of wine at the now-crystalline Ametis. The wine is said to have stained the crystal, transforming it into the stone we know as amethyst today.

Much in the same fashion, goblets of carved amethyst could deceive any who drank from them, for it would appear as though any water, or cheap wine, would be as dark and resplendent as the finest wine available. One could drink without end without intoxication. Charms in medieval lapidaries even include methods for sobering anyone who imbibed too much through the use of this crystal.

Amethyst as an archetype of temperance seeks to impart balance in the life of its student. The violet color of this crystal is often said to be of the highest spiritual frequency because it is the shortest wavelength, or highest energy, in the spectrum of visible light. Amethyst is overtly spiritual, and it is always seeking to unite us with our native connection with the divine presence that courses through all of creation.

Historically, the uses of amethyst ranged from the mystical and magical to the ecclesiastical. Amulets and talismans from ancient Egypt record the use of this stone from an early epoch. Later, amethyst was used by the faithful as a symbol of their devotion. Between the eleventh and fifteenth centuries, the Crusaders attached amethyst gemstones to their rosaries in order to represent faith in their mission, but also to ensure victory in battle.[2] In the Catholic Church, the tradition of gems of amethyst continues even today, as the stone is featured in the rings bestowed on bishops, cardinals, and occasionally in the Ring of the Fisherman, a signet ring worn by the pope. Amethyst was selected for use in these ecclesiastical gems because it served as a symbol of "piety and celibacy."[3] Those who undergo ordination must renounce the mundane world and its many seductive vices. This violet quartz also symbolizes chastity, and it has been suggested that it encourages marital fidelity, too.[4] Amethyst, having had a long history of being associated with sobriety, was a natural choice among those who were called to a clerical lifestyle not only because it exemplified the ideals of their path but also because its vibrations support and maintain a life free of indulgences. It was even recommended by the prophet Edgar Cayce that amethyst could be used for controlling one's temperament.[5] In helping to control one's overall disposition or behavior, amethyst can aid in eliminating behaviors that do not support your overall spiritual path and mental and emotional well-being.

Amethyst has achieved fame as a stone of temperance not only because of its relationship with wine. Energetically, the effects of amethyst are the result of two major functions of its crystalline frequency. First, amethyst, as the chief stone of the seventh ray, releases attachments, especially those that keep one encumbered in a state that prevents forward motion. Second, amethyst opens the flow of communication between the consciousness of humankind and the spiritual planes.

Amethyst and Limitations

In medieval lapidaries, amethyst's most popular use was to guard against inebriety while promoting wisdom, protection from evil, and victory on all fronts. Amethyst's ability to offer these benefits stems from its association with the violet ray, or purple ray, which is connected to spiritual attainment in modern gemstone therapy. The first step on the path to opening to Spirit is to release any attachments that inhibit the free expression of the divine within each of us.

Amethyst is "accessible and beautiful, gentle and works over a long period of time. It purifies, protects and strengthens divine connection, clearing out obstructions like addiction and over-thinking."[6] Oftentimes addictions manifest as a means of escapism or through a karmic pattern that has manifested in one's current life. Amethyst works to bring light to these scenarios such that they can be cleansed and completely resolved.

The violet ray, through amethyst, carries a message of release. Working with amethyst can help you release attachments and "let go of a past situation."[7] Amethyst can engender a sense of the spiritual in all matters because it awakens the inner ocean of wisdom and knowing. It stirs the intuition and provides understanding about one's limitations. Through the gift of perspective, this crystal offers an opportunity to resolve karmic ties and accept responsibility for our personal energies.

Temperance is not merely abstaining from the worldly vices. The archetype of temperance provides inner clarity and resolve to become an authentic person pursuing genuine spiritual growth. Drinking out of an amethyst vessel, on the one hand, is a declaration of purity in the face of temptation; on the other, it shows the desire to drink in the nourishment of Spirit in lieu of the licentiousness offered by the mundane world. By choosing the path of temperance, the spiritual seeker becomes a clearer channel for the spiritual forces. The intuition is clarified, even if only because there is less background noise in the mind. Temperance does not have to imply complete abstinence; instead, in this sense it is detachment from distraction. Amethyst's very nature is to remind one of what is holy, and this alone tends to promote distance from overindulgence.

Amethyst very often is used in crystal therapy as a means of breaking the bonds of addiction. As a model of temperance, amethyst can be employed in this manner because it treats the core of the issue. The essence of addiction is frequently one of transcendence: Addiction is a fixation on a substance, habit, or pattern that takes us outside of our normal consciousness. It is a misdirected attempt at achieving true spiritual transcendence, wherein the consciousness becomes acquainted with the divine. By opening the divine connection, amethyst creates a condition that overpowers the need for obsession or addiction. The intimate connection with the inner light casts away any shadows of negative mental habits. In color therapy, violet is used to "purify, disinfect, cleanse, and protect."[8] Amethyst is the most recognizable violet stone and it therefore utilizes these functions at both an inner and outer level when working with it, carrying it, or contemplating it. Amethyst is the gemstone that helps us meet and know our limitations, and in so doing we learn to trade them in for behaviors and thoughts that nourish us while we walk the spiritual path.

MEDITATION

RELEASING LIMITATIONS

Select a piece of amethyst to hold or wear for the following visualization. As you relax into a meditative state, imagine that your amethyst is growing in size until it is large enough to step inside. Follow the path into the heart of the stone, where you will find a sacred chamber with a cup carved from amethyst sitting on an altar. This is a sacred space for clearing away your limitations.

Now picture your most limiting beliefs, behaviors, and habits. Contemplate each one in turn and consciously decide whether you are ready to release these limitations in order to progress on your spiritual path. When you have made peace with these patterns that no longer serve you, take hold of the vessel carved from violet crystal sitting before you. Raise it over your head and pour its contents over yourself. Feel yourself being showered with clean, cool, crystal-clear water. As it washes over you, the energy of amethyst is carried by this sacred elixir and saturates every part of your being.

As the water runs down all parts of you, it breaks down the limiting patterns on each level of your existence. As you release these disharmonious frequencies they are replaced by a brilliant, violet light. Soon, your whole being is aglow with this amethystine radiance. Replace the cup on the altar, and it is refilled before your eyes. If you feel any stubborn limitations remaining, repeat the cleansing process as many times as you feel the need to. When finished, thank the consciousness of amethyst and return your awareness to your physical body.

Purified Spirit

In choosing temperance, one chooses a life purified through the action of the spiritual forces. The archetype of temperance results in fewer unhealthy attachments, fewer negative habits, and more focus on the metaphysical side of life. Amethyst supports all of these by clearing out limiting beliefs and by inducing a more serene state of being.

Amethyst is considered to be the spiritual stone extraordinaire for the lofty, peaceful energies that it imparts. This gemstone is an ideal ally in any tradition of sacred studies because it enhances the connection to the immaterial planes and purifies the mental bodies, thus facilitating communication with the higher self. Amethyst is the stone that can rapidly purify the inner landscape by simply turning the focus toward the celestial.

An element of sacrifice often accompanies this stage in spiritual unfoldment. When choosing to dedicate yourself to the path it becomes a necessity to let go of anything that holds you back from actually walking the path. Because of this, it is not uncommon for anyone who answers their spiritual calling to conquer bad habits, improve their thinking, and even to exercise moderation in food, drink, and other behaviors that can obstruct spiritual growth. Ultimately, these factors converge to provide the ideal situation for making positive changes in various avenues of life, from seeking a healthier diet, to selecting a cohort who supports one's spiritual direction. Anything that isn't aligned with this shift in frequency has a habit of falling by the wayside; for some, acquaintances fade into the past or careers may change.

The goal in this kind of transition is to engage in what Buddhists call the "Middle Way." Siddhartha Gautama, prior to becoming the Buddha, led a life that vacillated between extravagance and asceticism. He found that neither extreme was especially conducive to achieving self-actualization, let alone enlightenment, and so he outlined a path of moderation between the extremes of sensual indulgence and self-mortification. This, according to him, was the path of wisdom. For this reason Buddhists seek a path between the two extremes, for in this manner the body, mind, and spirit are equally nurtured and disciplined. Amethyst helps us cultivate the same level of moderation, by helping any extremes either fall away or be resolved through healing and transmutation.

The course of spiritual awakening and healing fostered by amethyst is one of purification. Only through the unfolding of inner cleansing can the initiate be ripe for entering the spiritual temple in which the innermost mysteries are revealed. Amethyst is a guide for engaging in the spiritual, mental, emotional, and even physical release that accompanies this leg of the journey.

AMETHYST AS AN ARCHETYPE:
THE VIOLET FLAME

Compared to most of the other archetypes in our odyssey through the mystery school teachings of the mineral kingdom, the violet flame is a relatively recent association. It is a spiritual tool for personal and planetary alchemy first revealed in the 1930s to Guy Ballard on Mt. Shasta, California, by a being who identified himself as the Comte de Saint Germain. The violet flame is a tool disseminated by the teachings of the ascended masters, particularly those of Saint Germain. Beautiful parables and stories describe the influence of these incorporeal teachers and the tools they provide us.

The purpose of the violet flame is to transmute any inappropriate or disharmonious thoughts, deeds, words, intentions, or karma in order to purify and prepare a spiritual practitioner for further unfoldment along the spiritual path.[9] The violet flame is considered to be carried on the seventh ray according to the teachings of Elizabeth Clare Prophet. In the esoteric teachings on the seven rays, the final, seventh, ray is the ray of ritual, magic, and alchemy, themes which transcend several systems on the seven rays. According to the authors Elizabeth Clare Prophet and Michel Coquet, it is symbolized by the color violet, or purple, and the seventh ray is carried by the amethyst gemstone.

The violet flame is a simple yet very effective tool. The basis of its application is to visualize violet fire in meditation or prayer. Frequently, decrees or mantras are chanted during this process in order to direct the energy of the violet flame. In recent years it has become commonplace to magnify and anchor the effects of this violet fire through the use of amethyst, among other gemstones.

Saint Germain bears the title "Master Alchemist." Amethyst, too, teaches the secrets of alchemy. Its quiet message is predicated on the basics learned from emerald, and then it goes further, but in a step-by-step manner. Amethyst has been connected to the spiritual realms since it first gained recognition by humankind. It works by gradually raising consciousness, allowing us to obtain true freedom.

The Universal Cleanser

In New Age crystal methodology, amethyst crystals are frequently employed to help cleanse and uplift other stones used in healing. A cluster of amethyst crystals is a useful tool, for other crystals can be placed on it to receive the healing light of the sacred fire that flickers within this violet gem. However, looking into the archetypal link, it becomes apparent that amethyst itself is not performing any cleansing on these other crystalline tools.

As an agent of the violet flame, amethyst holds the space for divine alchemy to transpire. Holding, wearing, or otherwise harnessing the activity of amethystine quartz provides all the resources necessary for transmutation, rather than cleansing. Amethyst does not sweep away accumulated energies in any situation; instead, its directive is to dispatch the properties of the seventh ray, including the violet flame, thereby raising the base resonant frequency of any energy stored within another crystal, or even in the ambient space around amethyst. This effectively makes use of the same principles as the archetype of temperance, wherein the violet flame seeks the underlying limitations of any situation and helps to release them from the overall pattern.

Amethyst works on both the inner and outer levels of manifestation in the universe. Principally, it begins its applications on the inner planes. Amethyst is generally felt at work in the mental, emotional, and spiritual levels before grounding its focus into the physical. Although its violet color is regarded as an overtly esoteric vibration, amethyst's color is, in fact, derived from iron, a metal with a very grounded essence. Iron brings the violet energy of amethyst into our bodily level of existence, carrying with it the changes it has effected, especially on the mental and spiritual levels.

Working with amethyst consciously in tandem with the violet flame magnifies the purifying, spiritualizing effects of this mystical stone.

While the initial archetype of temperance is largely an internal mechanism, the violet flame channels the same concepts from the microcosm to the macrocosm. Amethyst, through its sympathetic resonance with other members of the quartz family, can transmit the effects of alchemy far and wide, thus purifying and transmuting the causes and effects of disharmony on a global or even universal scale.

Water into Wine, and Other Miracles

Up until now the subject of alchemy has been investigated through the archetypes of emerald. Amethyst adds its own character to the alchemical arts, especially as a representative of the violet flame. In emerald one finds the guidebook of alchemy, the legendary emerald tablet, as well as the crucible in which it takes place, the Holy Grail. Amethyst serves as the sacred fire that burns beneath and around the grail stone; it is the fuel and the flame required for the Great Work to be successful.

Alchemy is a complex art, one requiring dedication, practice, and great patience to master. Amethyst helps the student of alchemy jumpstart his or her education through hands-on experience. Typically, learning to take the base metal—i.e., the "leaden" consciousness—and transfiguring it into gold is no easy feat. Amethyst works through the transcendent qualities of the violet flame to accelerate the foundation of alchemy.

In the ancient alchemical texts, descriptions of the fire beneath the cauldron or crucible extol the virtues of its intense heat. The inferno must be so hot that it can liquefy, sublimate, and otherwise transform the state of matter of a variety of compounds. Amethyst is the crystalline hearth in which this radiant blaze can be built. Connecting to its spiritual flame allows one to successfully perform feats of alchemy, for the violet flame is effectively a spiritual shortcut for transmuting the karma that has resulted from every thought, action, and lifetime we have ever experienced.

The violet flame is a tool not only for purifying but for enlivening our inner selves. Amethyst works in this same way to strengthen and crystallize our inner aspects, ultimately bringing them into manifestation in the here and now. The iron content, although minute, creates a corporeal, pragmatic, and earthy outlet for the otherwise nebulous, intangible nature of the immaterial planes. Because of this, working with amethyst enables one to begin to manifest latent talents and abilities that are otherwise considered to be psychic or supernatural.

Miracles are the natural order of the universe. Amethyst guides and educates the student of alchemy, teaching that the truth of miracles lies in their simplicity. Achieving transubstantiation of the wine and wafers into the Eucharist is an act reserved only for the clergy; however, the amethyst goblet allows for the deception of the world to fall away, leaving the miraculous act in the hands of any who choose it. Water into wine is effected simply by filling the amethyst cup. In this way, the paradigm of the supernatural slowly dissolves, and the student of the crystal mysteries is left viewing all mystical phenomena as the normative state.

Amethyst has been credited for helping people achieve gifts of prophecy, clairvoyance, lucid dreaming, and enhanced meditative states. Miracle cures, wisdom beyond earthly knowledge, and even breaking curses are possible with amethyst, according to traditional sources. Since amethyst abolishes limitations to spiritual actualization, this crystal enables its co-creator to attain spiritual gifts and talents solely by seeking the divine connection. Seeking the talents for their own sakes as novelties demeans the purity and innocence of miracles; alternatively, the power of amethyst is to release even the egoic attachment to the miracles themselves. They become second nature, an expression of inner and outer alchemy.

Finally, the effects of these miracles manifest as we release our burdens of fear. Virtually all limitations are expressions of fear, which stem from the ego and not from the true self. The violet flame is an unthinkably simple tool for stripping fear of its power through transmutation. Calling on its effects, or even utilizing amethyst crystals, can engender a loss of fear as it shifts into love. Amethyst is a humble, gentle stone, and it transmutes our fears and limitations into freedom.

Liberty and Justice for All

Amethyst has a unique relationship with the concept of liberty. For one thing, amethyst works through its archetype of temperance in order to release the bonds of addiction and overindulgence, thereby liberating the person from the effects of these scenarios. The action of amethyst is one that seeks out limitations in all forms; because of this, its energy can be viewed as a kind of missile that hones in on the bonds that hold us back. The work of amethyst is focused on freedom, both inner and outer.

In the ascended master teachings, Saint Germain is assigned the role as *chohan,* or steward, of the seventh ray. It is this ray that is in effect as the governing force of the current Aquarian Age. His role is to "deliver to the people of God the dispensation for the seventh age and the seventh ray—the violet ray of freedom, justice, mercy, alchemy and sacred ritual—a new lifewave, a new civilization, a new energy."[10] Amethyst allows the alchemy of the mineral kingdom to grow; emerald's role is largely that of personal transmutation, while amethyst widens the scope to include all of the beings of our world.

Connecting with the energy of the violet flame, especially through amethyst, is a fitting tool for instilling justice and freedom. These two energies manifest as the products of alchemy. When disharmonious energy is subjected to transmutation, it yields a state of grace through purification. The violet flame does not seek to sweep away negativity; instead it recycles it and leaves a situation with a renewed, positive influence. When the practice of spiritual alchemy is applied to group consciousness, injustice becomes decency and limitation becomes freedom.

The power of the violet flame is meant to pave the way for the highest path of human consciousness. As our leaden state becomes the transcendent, golden state of being, amethyst lights the path with freedom's flame. As the indomitable human spirit reaches new heights, amethyst readies it for the next step. For this reason, amethyst became one of the most indispensable healing stones during the inception of the current crystal movement. Decades ago it was one of the highest vibrations available to crystal therapists and lightworkers because it was needed to pave the way for our current progress.

The power of the violet flame is strengthening as well as refining. Glass, metal alloys, even foods can be tempered through the fiery power of heat. *Tempering,* a word that shares a root with *temperance,* provides an existing substance with additional fortitude. By tempering one's behavior, such as avoiding or releasing addictions or negative mental patterns, the end result is a stronger, clearer mind and body. Temperance and transmutation ready us to enter the spiritual sanctuary of the Age of Aquarius.

MEDITATION

INVOKING THE VIOLET FLAME

The violet flame is a life-changing tool that requires no props. All that is necessary is your intention, coupled with visualizing a violet fire wherever and whenever you choose to invoke the violet flame. Holding an amethyst while co-creating with the violet flame will amplify its effects, as well as provide additional focus for the mind and spirit of the practitioner.

Begin by cleansing the crystal with whichever method appeals to you. Hold it in your nondominant hand, and bring it to the heart center. Imagine breathing in through the stone, directly into your heart. With each breath you nourish and enliven the flame of your heart. Visualize it growing larger and blazing with a beautiful violet radiance.

Now, place the amethyst in your dominant hand and picture the violet fire of your heart traveling down your arm and through the amethyst. It can now be directed to any place, situation, or people requiring the transformative properties of the seventh ray. Continue sending the violet flame while envisioning any disharmony being transmuted into accord, chaos into order, distress into peace, and illness into radiant health. When complete, bring your awareness to your present location; thank the crystal for its participation and open your eyes.

Many books and articles discuss innumerable variations on the violet flame, such as affirmations, prayers, meditations, and visualizations. Try combining the use of amethyst with your favorite technique in order to amplify and cohere the intention.

AMETHYST AS AN ARCHETYPE: THE SANCTUARY

This stately and sacred jewel has attained a special place among stones of religious importance. Amethyst has been celebrated for its connotations of celibacy, sobriety, and all forms of purity, in sources both secular and sacred. The spiritual nature of amethyst is its most celebrated characteristic; it is noted for enhancing all types of mystical and metaphysical endeavors. Working consciously with amethyst almost certainly has the effect of spiritualizing your daily life; it helps you find sanctuary amid the mundane.

Amethyst has maintained ecclesiastical uses in many locations around the world. It has adorned the altars in Christian churches as well as the insignia of its clergymen.[11] In early Christian lapidaries this stone was representative of deep devotion, such as that experienced while deep in prayer, secluded from the world. Amethyst is touted as providing serenity and spiritual growth, much like time spent cloistered away can achieve.

In many of its forms, amethyst has been described in terms that evoke places of worship. As an example, let's consider the massive geodes of amethyst known as "cathedrals," commonly found in Brazil and Uruguay, although they are also present in other locations such as Mexico and Japan. Many times amethyst crystals are found as a drusy lining within a hollow rock cavity, properly known as a *vug*. These can be round or nearly spherical, in which case they are termed *geodes,* which are named for the round, Earth-shaped appearance of the rock before it is opened. Larger, more elongated vugs are known as "cathedrals," since their inner appearance and splendor is reminiscent of the inner sanctum of a Gothic cathedral. These specimens can range from a few inches tall to being large enough to stand within. In fact, there are specimens that are large enough to step into.

Amethyst cathedrals, especially large ones, command one's attention. They are as dramatic and breathtaking as an actual Gothic cathedral. The energy of these formations radiates a calm, tranquil peace throughout the air of the space in which they are installed. For this reason, they have found their way into the sacred spaces of many people, from the rooms of solitary meditators to communal places of worship. More than one church has used crystalline druses of amethyst to create spaces that are simply resplendent. The local Buddhist temple near my home has incorporated two symmetrical halves of an amethyst vug into its stunning central altar.

Another noteworthy formation of amethyst, called a "lightbrary," is found most commonly in Bolivia, and occasionally in Mexico and Japan. These crystals are among the largest specimens of single crystals of amethyst in the world; they can weigh many pounds and they set the record in size for a single crystal of amethyst. They exhibit a formation of parallel growth wherein there are numerous minute crystals growing parallel to the central crystal point. Each of the faces of the small crystals resembles the spires of a complex, towering cathedral. Although this crystal shape is more typical in other members of the quartz clan, it does occur with amethyst, too.

These crystals are sacred tools. Their distinctive name was coined by crystal healer Katrina Raphaell as one of the twelve master crystals; it "represents both a place where God is acknowledged (a cathedral) as well as a site of knowledge and learning (a library)."[12] They are radiant and often exhibit a quality of candescence, in which they appear to be lit from within. Crystals of this type are anchors of "the pure substance of undefined thought," and they hold sacred space around them.[13] They are potent crystalline tools that initiate intimate connection with the realm of sacred studies that recognizes the divine in all things.

The Greek myth of the nymph Ametis is encoded with information on how amethyst can connect us to sacred space. Recall that Ametis was a devotee of the goddess Artemis, and was en route to her shrine when her journey was interrupted by Dionysus. Artemis heard Ametis's pleas for help and saved her from harm by transforming her into crystal. When Dionysus poured the contents of his cup onto the stone, it is sometimes described as an act of rage, yet other interpretations regard it as a sobering libation, an offering to the being that he nearly hurt. The story of Ametis offers the hope of refuge from harm when we are devotional. Amethyst not only invokes a spiritual atmosphere, it evokes holiness and sanctity from the depths of one's being. When working with amethyst, ego, fear, and attachment fall by the wayside in order to make room for beatitude. The energy of this crystal prepares us for the miracles that come with grace and piety.

Building the Temple

Amethyst challenges the student of spirit to gradually shift his or her attention from an inward to an outward focus. While the preceding gemstones work on the inner planes and are suited to self-therapies, amethyst begins to widen the sphere of influence to the surrounding area. Placing amethyst in your personal space endows that space with an ambience of holiness and tranquility. This stillness permeates all who enter, not merely the owner of the space.

This violet member of the quartz family has a long history of use in building holy places. In the Book of Revelations, the city of New Jerusalem is described as displaying many gems. Among the most important of these stones are the twelve used in the foundation of the city. Although translations of this biblical passage vary significantly, the final stone is virtually always acknowledged as being amethyst. This twelfth stone of New Jerusalem, amethyst, is the gem that completes the spiritual retreat. Amethyst figures into the symbolism of New Jerusalem because of its connotations of piety, strength, and temperance. Furthermore, in archaic times amethyst was said to rid its owner of the woes of sorcery and evil. Amethyst would be the crowning stone of the New Jerusalem because it exerts such a benevolent, sanctified power, as well as because it would open the hearts and minds of all who would enter the city to embrace the immanence of divinity.

Amethyst has been cited as being crucial to the inception of the New Age awareness of crystals.[14] This may well be due to its ability to ignite the spark of awareness in all who work with it. Amethyst helps to shift the inner spiritual focus outward, thus urging its co-creators to spread love and serenity in their community and beyond. Amethyst helps all who connect to it with managing the impetus to grow the community. To do so, the temple must be built in order to foster our collective growth.

The work of amethyst may begin subtly, but as it purifies our inner and outer nature it makes way for the creation of sacred space. Whether it be a center of healing or meditation that uses amethyst to maintain an environment of purity, or whether it is worn by those seeking fulfilment through the mystical amid the everyday, amethyst serves to clear and align our paths and unite the efforts of like-minded souls toward begetting sacred space.

The inner structure of amethyst is characterized by an intergrowth of right- and left-handed quartz, as already described. When exposed to polarized light, this can reveal the optical effect referred to as Airy's spiral. These spiraling patterns encoded in amethyst's structure seem reminiscent of the shape of a labyrinth. The nature of the labyrinth, as found in Gothic cathedrals and medieval churches, is symbolic of the spiritual path. The labyrinth motif is representative of pilgrimage, spiritual growth, ecstatic rites, and other magico-religious ideas. Walking the labyrinth is a practice that has been adopted by some churches as well as by modern-day seekers as a means of achieving altered states of reality or for enhancing contemplation of the journey of the soul toward God. Because this labyrinthine pattern emerges from the core of amethyst, this stone can enable one to walk each and every step as though it were as contemplative and intentional as walking the holy maze.

Amethyst extends its violet energy to the area around it, and when worn can help one to engender more presence and awareness in the now. Amethyst permits a glimpse of Creator along every step of the path because it brings an awareness of the holiness of Earth as a temple. By deeply and intimately connecting to amethyst it is possible to embrace the holiness and beauty in your personal temple through dedication and commitment to the path.

MEDITATION

ENTERING THE TEMPLE

Amethyst cathedrals are eye-catching geodes lined with violet-colored crystals. They evoke an air of sanctity and peace wherever they are. For this meditation, any amethyst can be used for contemplation, although you may enjoy it best with a cathedral of any size. If such a specimen is unavailable, try the following exercise with a small cluster of amethyst.

Loosely gaze into the amethyst before you; allow your eyes to become unfocused, with the stone in front of them. Picture the amethyst growing larger until you can step inside the opening of the geode. At this point, let your eyes close completely and imagine yourself walking into the crystal.

You follow the opening along a corridor lined with amethyst clusters, and it leads you to a massive, crystalline church or temple. The cathedral is built entirely from amethyst, and every surface glitters. Reverently walk to the far end, where you will find an altar. Kneel before the altar with your hands in prayer position.

At this stage, you may offer prayers for any intention. If no specific needs come to mind, pray for the upliftment of Earth and all thereon. Afterward, stand up and return to your waking consciousness by following the path that led you to the cathedral. When you are ready, open your eyes.

Custodians of the New Earth

The violet ray is the frequency leading the evolutionary cycle of the Aquarian Age. Amethyst serves as a guide and anchor for this energy on our planet, all the while making it more accessible to those who live here. As the stone of the sanctuary, amethyst crystallizes the innate sacred presence of a space in order to maintain its integrity. It is in these sacred spaces that the seed of evolution incubates and grows.

Those who connect to the frequency of amethyst are supported by the virtues of the seventh ray, which oversees ceremony and ritual. In our sacred spaces, amethyst inspires its co-creators to engage in a personal practice whereby our body-mind-spirit is continually refined. The activity of the violet flame, one of the offshoots of the violet ray, also serves to refine and prepare the self and the planet for transformation. As these mechanisms within amethyst engage in the alchemical arts, the net resonant field of Earth and all who dwell here is fine-tuned. This subtle and gradual effect results in the final stages of preparation of the spiritual aspirant for the next level in his or her growth. Consciously co-creating with amethyst cultivates an awareness of where the earth is gradually headed. Amethyst encourages those of us on the forefront of these changes to take ownership of the evolutionary processes unfolding. In this way we can serve as leaders, teachers, prophets, and guides. Our personal sanctuaries become the point in which the new consciousness is moored to the third dimension.

Without negative attachments and limitations holding us back, the mind is better able to maintain diligence and reverence on the journey to recognizing wholeness. Amethyst is a superb teacher for learning to hold the space all around us through every step of the journey. As it raises our consciousness and transmutes disharmonious energies, amethyst reminds us that the scope of sanctuary is not limited by a perceived boundary of personal space. By tapping into the spiritual potential inherent in all places, amethyst helps us build the outer temple through the inner sanctum, a continuous observance of the devotional state of mind.

While in the beginning amethyst can help to clearly delineate the boundaries of one's personal sanctuary, the confines of that space will grow with the expansion of consciousness. What is initially a stopgap between the sacred and the secular is progressively opened and widened until it encompasses a greater expanse. Amethyst encourages the student of the mysteries to become responsible for his or her own energies and for those of others they come in contact with. The archetypes of amethyst endorse custodianship, first by releasing the limiting patterns that impede it, and later through the purification and transmutation of greater and greater areas. Truly, the perimeters of the personal sanctuaries will eventually overlap until a singular, global cathedral, one that envelops the whole world, is born.

In addition to pushing out beyond the range of previous limits, amethyst prepares its students in several other ways. When connecting to the archetypes of amethyst to promote planetary healing through the violet flame, one becomes a steward of the planet during this time of need. In return, amethyst prepares those working with it by helping them manifest the qualities that will be native to the denizens of the global temple. Clairvoyance, lucid dreaming, enhanced meditative states, and other spiritual gifts are the result of stepping into the role of leading the spiritual evolution of our world.

Stepping out into the world as if all land is holy land is the primary act in this co-creative undertaking. Dedication to the archetype of the sanctuary requires responsibility and discipline. It begins through preparation of the self, through temperance, and by externalizing that act of purification with the violet flame. As a result, more and more people will awaken and exhibit the same deference. The reward is an environment in which miracles become the normative state, and the supernatural becomes quite simply the natural.

EXERCISE
___

CREATING SANCTUARY

The following exercise is a loose outline meant to serve as inspiration for your own sacred space. You will need a flat surface to serve as the focal point or altar for your personal sanctuary. It can be permanent or temporary depending on the needs of your environment and lifestyle. You can select a fine piece of amethyst as the basic focal point, meant to serve as the anchor for your personal temple. A large terminated crystal, polished or natural, or a cluster or geode, also work well. Consider placing small pieces of amethyst in the four corners of the room in which your altar is located in order to maintain a purified environment for it. Enhance your sacred space with candles, incense, sacred art and images, healing music, or any other tools you desire.

When you have constructed your personal sanctuary, cleanse it by invoking the power of the violet flame to transmute any disharmonious energies remaining. To do so, simply visualize violet fire permeating your sacred space. Hold the intention that it will eliminate disharmony and provide you with transmuted, positive energy in its wake. If you have a favorite decree or affirmation for connecting to the violet flame, you may also speak it aloud. Sit, stand, or kneel before your altar and fold your hands together in prayer at the heart. Choose a prayer, affirmation, or visualization that supports your spiritual path. As you recite this, envision your sacred space filling with violet light; it grows brighter with every recitation or visualization.

When the physical confines of your temple have been filled with light, imagine that the boundaries stretch outward. They now extend beyond your personal temple to fill your home, your neighborhood, your town. Continue to affirm your intention and pray that it will benefit all sentient beings as it raises the collective consciousness of Earth. When the violet energy has encircled the globe, focus on peace, healing, and love. When you are ready, return your awareness to the room around you and express gratitude to amethyst for helping to anchor the positive changes.

AMETHYST IN CRYSTAL HEALING

In recent decades amethyst has enjoyed a sustained popularity among mineral collectors and crystal healers alike. Its rich shades of violet, the variety of its crystal forms, and the relative abundance of amethyst make it a perennial favorite. It has enjoyed the status of being a quintessential and versatile tool for effecting healing and transformation as well as one that supports the ongoing evolution of consciousness on Earth. Ancient myths and medieval lapidary manuscripts describe the spiritual virtues of amethyst, and modern compendia of crystals never seem to omit this important healing gemstone.

Physically, amethyst provides an infusion of energy to enhance the healing of any situation. It obtains its color from minute traces of iron, and this metal has a grounding, strengthening effect on our physical bodies. Some ancient sources ascribe a fiery energy to amethyst, and it shares the qualities of other stones governed by Mars in these texts: protection from bodily harm, victory in battle, and renewed strength. Amethyst can be used to provide spiritual support to any endeavor that may require endurance.

This violet form of quartz is occasionally recommended for stomachache and indigestion. It may be placed topically on the body for relief of such problems. It may also encourage healthy division of cells, thus facilitating recovery from any disruption in the growth of healthy cells, including broken bones, tumors, acne, or other forms of tissue degeneration or malformation.[15] It makes for an excellent adjunct to conventional allopathic therapies to restore cells to normal health and induce routine mitotic division.

Because its violet color is associated with the higher chakras, amethyst is often used for the health of the head and nervous system. Frequently prescribed for headaches, amethyst harmonizes the energy of the higher centers of the body and helps to channel them in a manner that integrates lovingly with our physical vessels. It can also help the brain and nervous tissues to regenerate after injury. Some sources also indicate that amethyst can be applied to improve the function of the endocrine system, especially for the control of blood sugar levels.

At the mental-emotional level, amethyst seeks to overcome limitations and attachments that impede development. The nature of amethyst's archetypes ensures that this stone can strengthen one's resolve to conquer negative habits and addictive traits. It helps to release the attachment to any vibration that is too dense or impure, thereby helping to shift attitudes toward balance and moderation.

It is a peaceful stone that can ameliorate states of unease and distress. "Amethyst's gentle persuasion temporarily stills the mundane thought processes that usually inundate the consciousness so that the mind can experience tranquility. Amethyst guides the awareness away from self-centered thought patterns as it lures the mind toward a deeper understanding."[16] It is calming enough to overcome most stress-related illnesses by addressing their cause while offering a provisional relief from symptoms, too.

Amethyst is a stone for clear thinking and developing trust. It bridges the mental and spiritual realms by facilitating recognition of the divine presence in perpetuity. Amethyst reduces the attachment to ego, which is itself a limitation experienced through the human state, and it makes room for keeping sight of the divine spark within. This musters confidence and strength, especially strength through surrender.

Amethyst is frequently associated with the expression "let go and let God." By releasing and transmuting attachments and other deleterious aspects of life, amethyst enlarges the portion of the consciousness that is focused on spiritual awareness. This greater awareness often results in more peace, serenity, and hope. Doubt and fear are displaced through certainty and discipline.

Spiritually, amethyst is an excellent stone for achieving humility. It helps to maintain the prayerful state, such as that experienced in a beautiful cathedral or temple. Crystals of amethyst inspire wisdom and develop intuition. Wearing amethyst "stirs the intuition" and "helps your mind become aware of its own intuitive aspect and, ideally, of that which lies just beyond it—soul itself."[17] It is a gemstone that opens the doorway to spirit; it can awaken memories of pure spirit and provide the impetus for dedication and diligence in metaphysical endeavors.

Amethyst is a versatile healing tool. Its myriad forms specialize its energy in a variety of ways, making it suitable for personal and environmental applications. Adding several pieces to your healing toolbox readies you for any number of situations in which it is useful, and it will often have untold benefits beyond just healing and overcoming personal challenges.

Varieties of Amethyst

Amethyst Cathedrals (Geodes)

Amethyst cathedrals are the ideal helpers for maintaining sacred space. One of the chief benefits of amethyst is its ability to cleanse and purify. The sheer size of many cathedral specimens can be breathtaking, but their energetic presence also uplifts the space in which they are kept. Their gleaming interiors are akin to the radiance of the violet flame continuously burning to remove negativity through the alchemical process of transmutation. For this reason, they are suited to healing spaces, meditation rooms, temples, and similar sacred spaces. The mass of the amethyst within them awakens the presence of Spirit among all who encounter them.

The crystal morphology referred to as "cathedral" will also be covered in the following chapter on quartz crystals.

Amethyst Cluster

While not strictly speaking a separate variety of amethyst, this formation is found in abundance and is easy to find in your favorite crystal shop. Clusters, caves, and cathedral-like geodes are excellent tools for harmonizing and transforming the energy of any space. Because amethyst clusters radiate the violet energy of the seventh ray in all directions, they purify and transmute energies on a broader scale than individual stones. They can also be harnessed for cleansing and empowering other crystals, jewelry, or sacred items. Clusters are especially effective for creating localized connections to the violet flame that burns in perpetuity for ongoing cleansing and spiritual support.

Clusters of appropriate size can also be used as a handheld healing tool. They may be used to sweep or comb the aura in order to "scrub" away negative attachments, residual energies released during healing, or to realign the layers of the aura if they are otherwise out of balance. These are versatile tools that enhance any crystal toolbox.

Ametrine

Part violet amethyst, part golden citrine, this colorful gemstone is a study in contrasts. Typically found in Bolivia, but also in Brazil, ametrine results from a process of twinning known as "Brazil Law twins." Effectively, this occurs when the lattice of the crystal reverses its crystallization direction partway through the growth of the stone. This may occur several times during the formation of some ametrines.

Citrine is a sister stone to amethyst, since it is also quartz colored by trace amounts of iron. Only in rare circumstances do they occur together naturally, although ametrine can also be artificially induced by uneven heating of amethyst crystals. Combining the golden, success-oriented energy of citrine with the violet ray of amethyst yields a unique stone that is capable of removing obstacles and empowering its user to achieve success in one swift motion. Ametrine can also balance the intuitive and more rational parts of our minds, helping each to understand the other better. One of its best uses may be to achieve equilibrium between spiritual and worldly pursuits; it is an excellent teacher for those needing to learn to accept that wealth and success on a mundane level are not mutually exclusive with spiritual growth.

Bancroft Amethyst and Auralite-23

These related amethysts are all found in Bancroft, Ontario. They feature inclusions of iron oxide (most commonly found as hematite), chevron growth patterns, and interesting color combinations. One classic locale for these crystals is Thunder Bay, where the crystals range from pale lavender to a deep, grape-jelly purple. Often these crystals may be found with a layer of hematite just below the surface of the crystal, resulting in an attractive "red cap," as they are commonly called.

The additional iron content of these formations of amethyst enables them to work more effectively on our lower chakras and more earthly levels of existence. The red-tipped specimens are especially effective for initiating the flow of kundalini energy from the base chakra to the crown center. They are also "well-suited to use for transmuting negativity in toxic environments."[18] The lighter amethysts from Thunder Bay, especially those that form in complex pockets of druse in white quartz, are excellent tools for cleansing the aura. They can also open us to the angelic presence and feel as though they help us spread our own wings.

Auralite-23 is purported to contain at least twenty-three other accessory minerals and elements as trace inclusions within its composition. Auralite comes in many color combinations, and nearly all of them contain chevron bands. In addition to the general properties of the red-tipped amethyst, auralite crystals have several unique characteristics. They are found in bedrock that formed 1.1 billion years ago, and while the auralites themselves may in fact be younger, this ancient, stony womb may account for their ability to tap into the Akashic records.[19] To me, they also exhibit a close connection to the violet flame. Overall, these are dynamic crystalline tools that act as sources of spiritual fire for transmutation, healing, and freedom.

Baobab Amethyst

The Baobab amethyst is so named for its origin in the Baobab Mine of Kenya. These crystals have only recently been made available, and they form in attractive crystal habits. Many of these stones are scepters and elestials (small crystals grown on the rhombohedral faces of a greater crystal), while some contain pockets of water and air trapped within.

The Baobab amethyst is an especially luminous crystal. Its color is frequently zoned, with darker patches highlighted by paler areas beneath. This African amethyst "joyfully focus[es] on linking you and all your experiences with spirit."[20] The complex elestial pattern in which most of these stones appear is thought to be a master emotional healer. The elestial crystal purges repressed emotions, while amethyst brings its power of transmutation. This makes for a powerful healing tool. The Baobab amethyst also teaches patience, kindness, and hope. They are reservoirs of divine wisdom and spiritual strength.

Chevron Amethyst

Chevron amethysts are among my favorites. They form as bands of pale and dark amethystine quartz in chevron, or V-shaped, layers.

Occasionally, bands of white and clear quartz or strata containing red hematite inclusions are found. It is available in masses as well as single crystals and clusters.

Chevron amethyst contains a wide spectrum of violet energies. It addresses deficiencies in the violet ray in multiple areas of life simultaneously, which can yield rapid results when compared to some other varieties of amethyst. Chevron amethyst also has a strengthening and fortifying effect; it roots us deeply on our path and assists in locating reserves of inner strength when confronted with challenges. It is especially effective in goal-setting. Using chevron amethyst attunes the violet ray to the many layers of the aura, thus releasing fears and limitations while gaining insight and perspective as we strive to grow.

Lavender (Cape Amethyst)

Lavender quartz, occasionally called "cape amethyst" or simply "lavender," is a semitranslucent, massive variety of amethyst. It rarely forms in transparent, well-formed crystals. Fine examples of this quartz can vary in transparency, with cloudy patches alongside clearer ones. Oftentimes it will be peppered with refractive areas resembling rainbows.

Lavender quartz promotes alignment on all levels. When we feel disconnected from Source, from our purpose in life, or from our intuition, lavender makes an excellent choice to get back on track. It can enable a deeper awareness of the spiritual nature of any circumstance or event in life, as well as promote better communication among the levels of your multidimensional self. Use lavender quartz for joint health, for its association with alignment can calibrate the components of the joints and alleviate any pain associated with them. Lavender can also support the integration of other crystals and tools, thus enabling them to have a more profound and synergistic effect on the human energy field.

Spirit Quartz

Spirit quartz is found in Boekenhout, Republic of South Africa, and is sometimes called "cactus quartz" because its morphology resembles this desert plant. It is named after a South African cleaning product called Spirit whose violet color is the same as that of the crystal. Spirit quartz forms as an even overgrowth of drusy crystals radiating out from a central crystal; they grow perpendicular to the central axis of the main point. These are traditionally collected and excavated on tribal lands by groups of indigenous women.[21] Spirit quartz varies dramatically in color, from amethyst to shades of citrine, smoky, white, and rose-colored quartz. The properties vary slightly in each variation or combination of colors, so the amethyst ones only are addressed here.

Spirit quartz is a multidimensional and multidirectional healing stone. Its energy can be focused or concentrated with the direction of the point, although when left at rest it also diffuses energy in all directions, much like a crystal cluster. Spirit quartz promotes group harmony; just as the small points grow together in harmony around a larger crystal core, this stone encourages individuals to work together for co-creating a common goal or purpose, much like the way this crystal is traditionally collected. This quality makes it an excellent aid to spiritual study groups or workshops that focus on spiritual practices and the healing arts. Similarly, amethyst spirit quartz can be used in meditation to "provide insight into family and community problems."[22]

These unique crystals are exceptionally capable of magnifying energy. Use them to charge and magnify other stones, to cohere separate energy toward a common purpose, or to attract more energy to fuel a specific idea or objective. The number and size of the crystals along the faces of the crystal body are proportionate to the ability of these minerals to magnify and intensify.[23]

Vera Cruz Amethyst

Amethyst crystals from Vera Cruz, Mexico, exhibit elongated prism faces unlike specimens from many other locations. They tend to have a brilliant, vitreous luster and excellent clarity despite the fact that their color is often paler than many other amethysts. Some crystals, which tend more toward a medium-purple color, exhibit the characteristic Muzo habit and horizontal striations consistent with Lemurian seed crystals typically found in Brazil (see chapter 6), as well as many of the attributes of Lemurian crystals.

Vera Cruz amethysts are breathtakingly radiant. They have a directional force to them lacking in many other amethyst gems. Their energy can help you connect to aesthetics, encouraging you to appreciate the beauty that is all around us.[24] They are luminous crystals, and they bring the energy of amethyst to a pure, pristine level. Placed around your home or used in grids, these crystalline tools hold the environmental energy at a cleaner and clearer vibration. Holding Vera Cruz amethyst during meditation links the heart and the crown centers. These stones are excellent allies for anyone working to heal planet Earth who is also working with Earthkeeper crystals, which are giant quartz crystals that act as the stewards and record keepers of the planet. Vera Cruz amethyst helps maintain a pure, temple-like environment around the Earthkeepers in order to help awaken their latent healing energies.

Related Stones

Lavender Quartzite

This gemstone is sold under several names, including lavender quartz and violet quartz, thereby conflating it with other closely related gemstones. It is a fine-grained, massive variety of quartz with a lavender or purplish gray tint; most pieces exhibit inclusions of other minerals, such as tiny flecks of mica. Lavender quartzite is found in Arizona.

Using this stone is a much gentler experience than its cousins amethyst and the true lavender quartz. It is much more grounding, and it connects readily to the earth. The earth-tone version of the violet ray that is present in this stone is nurturing, supportive, and motherly. Lavender quartzite supports the health of our physical structure, especially our bones, teeth, cartilage, and ligaments.

Purple Fluorite

Fluorite is chemically and structurally very different from the quartz family. Purple fluorite can, however, connect to the violet ray and serve as a bridge between the physical manifestations of that ray and the spiritual source of it. It helps to break down mental and physical barriers to the effects of the violet ray and therefore serves as an excellent adjunct to the energy of amethyst.

The cubic morphology of fluorite enables it to be more grounding than amethyst. It frequently crystallizes as cubes, octahedrons, and combinations of the two. These forms are very stabilizing; they also facilitate grounded, linear thought and promote self-discipline. Using fluorite can quiet the mind to permit the more spiritual nature of the violet ray, as carried by amethyst, to root itself more deeply within your being and your spiritual practice

Purple Tourmaline

According to some sources, amethyst's reign as the carrier of the violet ray is coming to an end.[25] In the 1980s, when information on gemstone therapy was becoming more widely available, it was written that amethyst would be succeeded by a stone already known on the planet, and that the violet ray would eventually transition from amethyst to its new steward.[26] Recently, that gemstone was unveiled, and it is purple tourmaline. The violet ray is still gradually transitioning from amethyst to tourmaline even now.

Purple tourmaline shares a crystal system with amethyst and is also a silicate. It contains lithium, among several other constituents, which accounts for its calming, soothing, and overtly spiritual influence. It is "connected with the highest spirituality and continually teaches us."[27] It works at a higher level than amethyst does; because of this, purple tourmaline seeks to assist its wearer in creating his or her own reality. This goes beyond the simple level of manifestation, as it actually helps you to reach and fulfill your goals on every level. It works to help you let go of the barriers that stand in the way of your achievements, and it transmutes them into helpful vibrations instead. It is an excellent stone for writers, and it also supports the health of the nervous system.

Ruby Lavender Quartz

Ruby lavender quartz, sometimes sold as pink lazurine, is a lavender-to-pink lab-created gemstone. Rumored to be the byproduct of scientific experiments, this material is rich in neodymium, which accounts for its characteristic color. In differing wavelengths of light, such as artificial lighting versus sunlight, this gem appears to change color from pink to purple. It is actually a fused quartz glass of optical or near-optical quality rather than a true crystalline quartz.

Ruby lavender quartz is strongly associated with the violet flame. Because it has a strong pink tinge even in its lavender state, this stone engenders a softer, more feminine energy than amethyst. It works closely on the heart center and the emotional body, especially with regard to instilling empathic protection from the world around its wearer. This makes it an excellent stone for anyone engaged in the healing arts, for it prevents the tendency to take on any energy or thought forms being released by a client. Additionally, as it channels the transmutation power of the violet flame, ruby lavender quartz also purifies energies that are released during healing.

Working with ruby lavender quartz also activates the high heart chakra. Known also as the witness point and the thymus chakra, this energy center is located between the heart and the throat chakras, and it is associated with higher, more spiritual expressions of love. The high heart chakra is also associated with the immune system. It is gradually evolving in all of humanity, and this stone facilitates the opening and strengthening of the higher heart. Ruby lavender quartz thus opens the heart and mind to deep levels of compassion, and it bridges the intuitive and emotional centers in doing so.

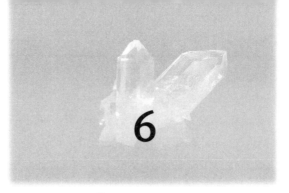

6

QUARTZ

The Wand and the Lens

Quartz is easily the most popular New Age gemstone. Tumbled stones, raw crystals, and faceted gems adorn almost every metaphysical student at one point or another. As one of the most abundant mineral groups, quartz is accessible on virtually every continent in one form or another. It has been considered to be the most important healing tool in the mineral kingdom, both for its availability and for its function.

While it is available in many variations, the archetypes of this chapter will largely focus on the clear, crystalline varieties of quartz. Apart from transparent crystals, well-formed specimens of quartz can be found in practically every color of the rainbow. Massive and microcrystalline types of quartz occur much more frequently than crystal habits, and they include the chalcedony group, such as agates and jaspers and onyx, as well as tiger eye, pietersite, flint, chert, and massive colored quartzes such as rose quartz and aventurine. Quartz is a major rock-forming mineral, and it is common in rocks such as granite, gneiss, sandstone, and others.

Quartz's name is derived from a Germanic root word of uncertain origin, and it has historically been referred to as "rock crystal," especially when gemmy and clear. Crystal itself comes from the Greek root word *krustallos,* meaning "frozen," referring to the ancient belief that quartz was a form of permanently frozen water. It is formed of silicon dioxide in its alpha state, and its morphology is generally six-sided. The hexagonal symmetry of this mineral results in beautiful crystal habits that can vary from one location to the next.

The physical, mechanical, and optical properties of quartz have been thoroughly explored. Quartz's technological and industrial applications frequently stem from its mechanical property of piezoelectricity: this means that when placed under stress, the lattice of the mineral is mechanically deformed, during which time the crystal generates an electrical charge. Quartz can similarly be used as an oscillator, such as those found in clocks and watches.

This mineral is considered an optically active material. Quartz polarizes incident light, which means that it coheres the waves of light that pass through it, as though the light has been aligned in a common orientation instead of a random dispersion. Quartz crystals also rotate the plane of polarized light when the light travels parallel to the central axis of the stone.

Centers of production for quartz mines in the United States include Arkansas, New York, Colorado, Georgia, and several other locations. Quartz is also found in Central and South American countries such as Brazil, Mexico, Uruguay, Bolivia, Colombia, and Peru, as well as in several African nations, a number of places in Europe, such as the Alps, and in Asia. Quartz is ubiquitous and is available in many categories of quality and color.

Constituting roughly 12 percent of the total mineral content of Earth's crust, quartz is abundant enough to have been universally available to premodern societies, even if it meant trading or traveling in order to acquire this precious commodity.[1] Before the advent of quality glassmaking, quartz's transparency and durability designated it as an auspicious and marvelous substance. Native cultures thought that crystals were the reincarnations of fallen gods, pieces of the sun, or even the dwellings of ancestors. Quartz's supernatural affiliations subsequently led to widespread acceptance of its powers to heal, control the elements, and command the powers of light.

In Asia, quartz has been esteemed as a precious substance on par with jade, gold, pearls, and ivory. Quartz is occasionally chosen as a special representation of the Hindu god Shiva, with the innate prismatic form celebrated as a natural lingam, the phallic icon of the Creator. Ritual implements carved from quartz can be found in many parts of Asia, including Japan, China, and the Himalayas; the nature of crystal as a luminous medium symbolized the potential for enlightenment.

Among Europeans, quartz, often called "rock crystal," was generally tied to lunar symbolism. Like the moon, it reflected ambient light while simultaneously conveying impressions of magic and mysticism. For this reason, quartz was frequently connected to the astrological sign Cancer and was used to heal any afflictions under the auspices of this sign. Quartz represented the mysteries of light and second sight. As lapidary arts grew more refined, court magicians and astrologers consulted crystal balls instead of communing with raw, unfashioned quartz.

Quartz was at the forefront of changing tastes in the art of carving gemstones. Sculptural carvings, functional tools, and jewelry all adapted the outward forms of quartz to suit shifting aesthetics. Rock crystal would persist into the technological age, where it is used in oscillators in watches, optical lenses, and reduced to silicon in furnaces for modern-day computing needs. Crystals, quartz and otherwise, surround modern life in well-hidden guises. When the shift in consciousness began during the crystal renaissance of the New Age, quartz was touted as the most important of all healing stones, a title it still carries. Admittedly, of all the stones that are part of this book, quartz is the most difficult to encapsulate, as its uses are practically innumerable.

QUARTZ AS AN ARCHETYPE:
THE WAND

Close your eyes and visualize a wizard or other magician. Though no two people have the same notion of what such a person looks like, many cannot separate the magician from his or her wand. For many people, elaborate wands tipped with crystalline points are the quintessential magical tools. Quartz, as a multidimensional manifestation and healing tool, is the perfect crystal wand. Its history from culture to culture includes many applications of its prismatic shape as a handheld ritual implement that empowers the bearer of a quartz crystal to shape the world.

Among the earliest recorded uses of quartz crystals, humankind has valued the mineral for its transparency and crystal form. Shamanic traditions use quartz in a number of ways. Crystals may be included in medicine bags and healing bundles, as well as worn as pendants, placed on the body of the sick, or even implanted beneath the skin. Above all these applications, however, the ceremonial use of crystal as the archetypal wand arises as the most recognizable and universal.

Crystal wands exist in many incarnations both ancient and modern. Earliest uses involve the addition of natural crystals to ritual implements as a means of imbuing them with spiritual power, or simply used in their own natural state. Wands and related artifacts can be found among Native American cultures and native populations of Europe and Africa. This concept was further refined, and later epochs would find more sophisticated crystal relics being crafted. A fine example of such a wand among Native Americans can be found in the Santa Barbara Museum of Natural History in California; it is a Chumash artifact.[2]

Scepters and crooks as well as other accoutrements with rock crystal components were used among nobility and the clergy. Among the Scottish crown jewels, for example, there is a royal scepter topped with a crystal orb that actually combines two of the archetypes of this gemstone.[3] Quartz maintained a special place in religious movements, as it symbolized light and enlightenment, and a crystal crook once belonging to an abbess in medieval France continues the tradition of the crystal wand.[4] Those who held such implements were the light-keepers and teachers of their time; they could disseminate and direct wisdom and virtue through their wandlike tools.

Natural forms of quartz with wand-shaped morphologies have become popular today. Laser wands, which are long and tapering, with minute crystal faces at the point, are coveted tools among healers and crystal therapists. The name *laser* denotes the intensely focused stream of energy that is directed through this kind of crystal. Scepter quartz, another type of wandlike quartz, is reminiscent of the symbol of power wielded by kings and emperors. They are crystals whose terminations are "capped" with another crystal, generally wider in diameter, giving them a phallic appearance.

As the fields of crystal healing and other therapeutic applications of minerals advance, new tools are always being innovated. Crystals can be shaped into precise forms, such as the Vogel crystals, which are double-terminated wands cut to precise angles, so-named for their innovator, research scientist Marcel Vogel. After Vogel's passing, several talented lapidary artists continued to evolve the designs, with new crystal wands being constructed to have specific spiritual benefits. And, of course, the classic wand, in copper or wood and topped with a crystal, is still being used by healers and magic-makers.

The wand is a symbol of power; it signifies command over the elements. Magicians of various traditions utilize different permutations of the wand as tools for directing, enhancing, and focusing their personal power and the energy of the universe. The wand is a projective masculine symbol. It is descended from common ancestral symbols scattered across the globe that share not only the outward form but also the underlying meaning of mastery.

The Divine Masculine Principle

In the mystery traditions, the cup and cauldron are representative of the feminine aspect of Creator, the Goddess. In perfect balance to these feminine, receptive forms, the wand arises as the masculine counterpart and consort to the Goddess. Quartz crystals are a prototypic form of the wand in that their tapering form yields an ideal tool for directing and focusing energy. Just as the chalice is symbolic of the womb, the wand evolved as a phallic motif that embodied the divine masculine.

By way of symbolism and sympathetic resonance, early religions and spiritual beliefs centered around daily life, and ritual became a means of requesting supernatural intervention on behalf of humankind. The cup and the wand, as representations of reproductive organs, share a heritage with the earliest fertility cults, and their use is dispersed throughout the world under many names and shapes. The overtly phallic nature of the wand may have originally meant to ensure virility among people, live-stock, and crops; soon, the act of using the wand to intercede magically would have encouraged its evolution into a stylized ritual tool.

The wand is closely linked to several other embodiments of the divine masculine or God archetype. It shares its procreative imagery with the Shiva lingam, a figurative icon of the Creator in Hinduism. Occasionally, the lingam can be a natural or polished quartz crystal referred to as a *spatika* lingam. Wands also share a heritage with serpent symbolism, inasmuch as the serpent is also used as a fertility symbol in many cultures.

The crystal wand, whether a natural formation or a work of art tipped with stone, is a descendant of the prototypical wand. Crystal wands continue the tradition of symbolic representation of the divine masculine, and they are complementary to the feminine principle seen in the emerald's grail archetype. Where emerald represents the chalice of the Goddess, the rock crystal is the masculine energy made crystal-line. Together, they unite in the Great Rite, a ritual symbolic of procreative union.

The wand balances its feminine polarity, offering outer strength, clarity, and direction alongside the energy of receptivity and regeneration that the grail brings. In connecting to the energy of the archetypal wand, quartz guides the spiritual practitioner to a place in which he or she owns up to both inner and outer strength. Quartz is traditionally viewed as a stone of amplification, and like the magical wand it amplifies and coheres the personal energy of its user. Quartz allows the walker of the spiritual path to synthesize all of the lessons from the preceding chapters and apply them outwardly.

Quartz as a wand is the tool that helps you to express your power. In some ways it resembles the warriorlike, pointed focus of the obsidian's first archetype, the spear. Even in composition, both quartz and obsidian are comprised of silica; however, quartz refines and rarefies the principles seeded by obsidian. The crystalline order that obsidian lacks is found in quartz in abundance. It is this very crystallinity that accounts for the spiritual properties of quartz crystals and yields the physical, optical, and mechanical properties that render them so useful in technology.

The wand is pointed, focused, and directional. It is used by the magician to concentrate his or her personal power in order to effect change in the outer world in accordance with changes made on the inner levels. The wand implies power; like the royal scepter or shepherd's crook, it is used to conduct energy. This inherent idea of movement and projection offers a counterpoint to the nature of the Goddess's vessel, which offers stillness and receptivity. With the wand, the walker of the spiritual path applies both personal and universal energies in order to create change.

The wand works through the will, which has been tempered and trained by the previous crystal archetypes. The wand applies the alchemical laws for worldly results, not just for achieving inner growth and healing. Because of this, quartz becomes the tool for integrating the inner and outer planes and for uniting the spiritual with the material worlds. By definition, this is the level of achieving spiritual mastery, wherein balance in all aspects of life has been achieved.

Taking this one step further, quartz has occupied such a pivotal role in crystal healing and spiritual growth because the connotation of movement, with which the wand is associated, can serve to imply evolution. Quartz has been used to facilitate positive changes, both personally and on a planetary level, because it literally points us forward, helping us achieve our next level of development.

The Prism

As light passes through a crystal wand, especially when found in its native form, it is broken into the full complement of colors in the spectrum. Quartz has held its place as a magical stone in many cultures because of its physical characteristics and because of its interaction with light. To ancient people these were mysterious, almost supernatural qualities, and they revered quartz crystals as spiritual tools imbued with metaphysical dominion over the physical world.

The way that quartz refracts light gives it an affinity to all of the seven rays in terms of both optical and occult rays. Quartz crystals are the most basic tools of crystal healing and gemstone therapy. They empower the healer to direct energy through them, which permits blockages to be removed and old patterns to be broken down and replaced. Simultaneously, quartz nourishes the whole being with all seven colors of vital energy. An invaluable tool, quartz "unifies the seven rainbow rays of the various gemstones and infuses the wholeness of White Light" into the recipient of the healing.[5]

The unity and coherence of energy that is transmitted by the crystal wand relates to similar principles of unity and cohesion among humankind. Many times quartz crystals will display beautiful, prismatic inclusions within. These rainbows result from pressure flaws within the quartz whereby damage or trauma creates a fissure or crack in the heart of the stone. Light plays on these beautifully yielding, brilliant, and colorful prisms. Katrina Raphaell, when speaking of rainbow crystals, writes that the "rainbow is a symbol of unity as it blends each color harmoniously with the rest, demonstrating for us how to embrace the elements in our life."[6]

Prisms teach us to see all aspects of life. The crystal wand, because it yields beautiful rainbows, conveys hope and inspires one to create change. The rainbows within crystals that are created as light passes through them "are a direct link from the earth into the ethers through which prayers, hopes, dreams and visions can traverse."[7] Shamans the world over have viewed the rainbow as a bridge between the different planes of reality. The prismatic form of the crystal wand furthers its celestial connections and functions as an intermediary between dimensions for the magician or healer. The wand, as a prism, may also have inspired early crystal mystics to further explore the archetypal connection between crystals and light.

MEDITATION

THE CRYSTAL WAND

Choose your most beloved piece of quartz for this meditation. It needn't be a crystal wand because the wand you'll work with here is a symbolic one held within the stone itself. Begin with a cleansed crystal and make yourself comfortable with your crystal held in your dominant hand.

Imagine that the crystal is growing in size; it becomes as large as a house. On the surface of the face nearest to you visualize a doorway or portal. You sense a gentle tug toward this opening, and you walk into the stone. Follow the corridor within until you come to a large room. In the center of this space there is a table, and a wand sits on it.

Walk up to the table and inspect the wand. What does it look like? From what materials is it made? Pick it up and feel it. Is it smooth? Is it heavy? When you hold it in your dominant hand, you feel the wand coming to life. It begins to hum and glow. Hold it before you and allow it to radiate its light to your entire being. Feel the power and strength that it imparts to you.

Next, direct the wand at your root chakra. Hold it there until this center is cleared and energized. Repeat this with each of the six remaining energy centers. When you have completed, return the wand to its place on the table. Retrace your steps and exit the stone.

When you return your awareness to your physical body, take several deep breaths before opening your eyes. Now repeat the exercise with the crystal that you hold. Compare results.

QUARTZ AS AN ARCHETYPE:
THE LENS

Natural prisms of rock crystal straightforwardly refract light into its components, thereby revealing a hidden spectrum available in white light. Among ancient peoples and in a tradition that continues to this day, the nature of quartz has been linked to light, both solar and lunar. The pristine clarity and utilitarian durability of quartz lends it to fashioning a variety of optical tools, and as time went by prisms soon gave way to the fashioning of lenses.

Examples of ancient optical technology have been systematically overlooked by most of the academic world, although traces of it are extant in many "primitive" cultures. Magnifying lenses, burning globes, and even lenses correcting for astigmatism have been found at archeological sites, with many other instances of optical imagery—such as the sun disc of the Egyptians, which was more than likely a depiction of a lens, and Japanese prism and lentoid carvings—found among quartz artifacts.[8] The role of quartz is to focus, just as a lens condenses light into a single point of focus. Consequently, the function of quartz, when polished and smoothed, cannot be separated from the ancient theology of light.

The Optics of Quartz

The word *crystal* evokes impressions of clarity and brightness. The optical nature of quartz is virtually inseparable from it at every stage in human history. Today's technology permits us to explore the mysteries of this mineral and its relationship with light in a way that is more than symbolic, however. Because of the arrangement of its constituent elements, quartz displays many properties that glass and other transparent substances do not. Quartz is considered to be an excellent medium for many applications in optics, for it exhibits a good dispersion of light, mild birefringence (the refraction of light in two slightly different directions to form two rays, known as "double-refraction"), and it even polarizes light.

When polished smooth, quartz becomes an excellent magnifier. Examples of plano-convex lenses (flat on the bottom and rounded on the upper surface), biconvex lenses (rounded on each side), and spheres of optical quality are extant at many archeological sites. Examples of such lenses that date back thousands of years may also be found in many museums today. Quartz was used by artisans to magnify their work in order to achieve fine details. Quartz was also used as sacred burning globes that condensed the sun's rays in order to start sacred fires. Further evidence suggests that eyeglasses and telescopes employed quartz lenses long before the dates originally posited by academics.

One of quartz's more noteworthy properties is its ability to polarize light. Polarization occurs in quartz because of its crystalline structure, as light moves along the axes of the crystal. The end result is an organized pattern in the waves of light passing through it; essentially the movement of light is no longer erratic or randomized, and it becomes coherent, as though the waves all line up with one another. Due to the structure of quartz, it exhibits a much rarer phenomenon during polarization, too. When light travels parallel to the central axis of the crystal structure, as if moving from base to tip, the light both polarizes and rotates. The moving plane of light thus becomes a luminous helix as it courses through the stone.[9]

In a number of myths and philosophies, quartz is intimately linked to the luminary bodies of the sky, the sun, and the moon. Spheres and other rounded shapes of quartz display extraordinary optical effects; even a small amount of ambient light can be magnified, thus appearing to light the stone from within. Cultures made use of quartz's sensitivity to light in order to create functional tools and even art. In Egypt, plano-convex lenses were used as the corneas of the eyes of statues, bringing a lifelike, lucent air to the figures. I have observed the same technique used to make the eyes of centuries-old statues in Japan, as well. Additionally, functional magnifiers and globes could be used for cauterizing wounds and igniting celebratory pyres.

The exploration of optics, when coupled with ancient attitudes about the role of light in the creation of the universe, engendered a theology of light, and rock crystal has been featured as an integral part of its imagery. One such illustration of this connection stems from the Orphic cult of ancient Greece, which was associated with literature ascribed to the mythical poet Orpheus, who descended into Hades and returned, and who was said to have invented the mysteries of Dionysus. "Fundamental to the Orphic cult is the image of a cosmic egg from which light and fire stream forth. The egg is obviously a crystal ball or glass water-filled globe," and from this crystal egg was born their creator god.[10]

The Bible mentions optical imagery, too, and in the vision of Ezekial, the throne of God is depicted as resting "on a sea of beautiful, sparkling, pure white crystal."[11] Is it possible that this "sea of crystal" in fact refers to receiving a vision through a polished lens or globe? It may, in fact, be a remnant of earlier sects of light theology, wherein the throne of God represents the cosmic source of all light. The connections between crystal and light are nearly universal. Scientist and "crystallographer" Frank Dorland writes that "somewhere in the background of most civilizations there is a legend about a magical crystal that illuminates, guides and protects people from evil."[12]

The Crystal Sun

Central to the worship of many people is the source of all life on our planet, the sun. The sun is responsible for light, warmth, and energy; it fuels the growth of plants, which in turn feed the other kingdoms of life. In short, without the sun, humankind would not exist. Philosophers and mystics have recognized this and sought to understand the nature and function of this celestial light.

Quartz spheres and lenses have been associated with solar and lunar bodies because of their excellent ability to collect ambient light. Even in environments with low lighting, a round, clear piece of crystal will appear to collect light from the surroundings, almost as if lit from within. This quality has served as an inspiration for the idea of the crystal sun, a concept once integral to the understanding of the cosmos.

The most complete surviving account of the crystal sun in antiquity comes from Philolaus, a Presocratic Greek philosopher often credited with originating the idea that Earth is not the central body of the universe. In his writings, the depiction of the crystal sun remains, although it has baffled many students of his writings. Essentially, Philolaus describes three suns, reflecting the once-widespread belief in a crystal sun responsible for collecting and distributing the light of the celestial spaces to the earth:

> The "three suns" described by Philolaos [Philolaus] are really two, the third being merely the light which travels to us by refraction. The "first sun" is the ambient light, and the "second sun" is the actual object of crystal which gathers it in and refracts it to us. Three suns should thus be really more properly expressed as "three stages of sunlight": (1) ambient light exists round the centre of the cosmos; (2) the crystal sun gathers it in and refracts it toward us; and (3) that refracted light then travels from the crystal body to the earth and our eyes.[13]

The crystal sun thus described becomes symbolic of the collection and distribution of the energies of the heavens and the rerouting, both literal and metaphorical, of the light toward the earth. This echoes the act of the creation of the world. The belief in the heavenly fire was reenacted through the lighting of sacred fires by using burning globes, a tradition once recorded by ancient Greeks that stretches back to ancient Vedic cultures.[14]

Crystal balls and orbs feature prominently in various cultures. In China and Japan they are often connected to myths of dragons, and the iconography of these countries frequently depicts dragons with crystal spheres and glowing, fiery pearls. The crystals there are preferred in polished forms. "Shaped like a globe, they represent the sphere of the earth, which the celestial dragon holds in its claws or between its jaws."[15]

Crystal balls can be found among many votive offerings and funerary goods, and they factor into such royal regalia as the Scottish Crown Jewels. These sacred objets d'art were also prized in pre-Columbian Mesoamerican cultures: the Aztecs called rock crystal *yztac tehuilotl,* meaning "round stones like drops of water."[16] The roundness of river-tumbled stones spurred the creation of polished ritual tools, perhaps including the famous crystal skulls, described later in this chapter. The holiness of quartz, rounded or not, was inseparable from the light-induced phenomena it conveyed. Some native cultures such as the Navajo "believe it is thanks to rock crystal that the sun first rose and illuminated the world," while shamans of Oceania believed crystals to be "stones of light" that were fragments of the celestial throne.[17]

Fire from Heaven

Quartz as a lens or sphere represents the descent of light into matter, just as the crystal sun directs light onto Earth. Quartz has been regarded as a mystical substance that can remain cold even as it brings light, warmth, and fire to whatever is placed below it. Quartz could seemingly make fire descend from the sky, as the light that passes through it can set kindling ablaze. This ability to make immaterial light into tangible flame is not unlike quartz's capacity to put one in touch with the spiritual levels of existence.

The act of spirit descending into earthly matter by means of a crystal orb is similar to the image of a cone of light being refracted by a sphere or lens and condensing down to a finite point. The action of the orb is to transduce ambient, discarnate light into physical embodiment, just as it gathers visible light via refraction. Science journalist Robert Temple has said that "the image of the descending soul as a cone of light being emitted from the 'crystal ball' or even 'mini-crystal sun' of its natural spiritual condition into the realms of matter preserves a tradition of deep metaphysical light-theology which ultimately derives from Egypt and was preserved in Greece by the mystery schools and the Neoplatonist philosophers."[18]

What we learn from the Pythagoreans and other learned men and women of ancient Greece is that "individual souls were envisaged as little crystal suns, emitting their own divine light and fire in cones downward into matter, in their process of reincarnation."[19] This is likely to have been carried over into later religious beliefs throughout Western Europe, and it would account for the great number of funerary globes and spheres that accompany the dead. Since the crystal sphere represents the descent of spirit into matter, the globes, which were placed with the remains of the dead, assisted the souls of the deceased in returning from material existence as they ascend toward the heavens.

Working with quartz fosters an intimate connection to holy fire, the divine spark of light and warmth that is within each person. The spiritual light from which we are all descended is akin to Creator, variously described as the cosmic light of the universe, the Great Central Sun, and the Source. Just as the crystal sun captures the essence of God and refracts it to fuel the planet, our soul's own metaphorical crystal sun is a lens that focuses the light of Source on a smaller scale, enabling a small spark of the Logos to become an incarnated individual being on planet Earth.

Quartz spheres and lenses, therefore, can be used to increase one's light quotient by drawing more and more light into one's being. There is a Celtic belief that suggests a similar concept; it is illustrated by a magnificent artifact called the *liath meisicith,* a magic brooch or buckle, in the center of which was a large quartz crystal, a feature of the ceremonial robes of the Druid priest. Though regarded as a magnifier or burning lens, this plano-convex quartz crystal was meant to draw down *logh,* or "heavenly fire," in ceremony.[20] Etymologically, all the ideas concerning the optics of quartz are intertwined; *light, Logos,* and *logh* all suggest a common origin, one that implies that our own relationship to the divine light cannot be ignored.

All of matter surrounding us is in constant vibration; much of it is actually empty space. Crystals, for all their solidity and firmness, are also in constant flux. If you could magnify everything enough, solid matter begins to resemble the wave particles of which light is comprised. A friend of mine put it best in a conversation: all matter is simply light slowed down. Quartz, as the lens or crystal sun, focuses the immaterial light into the material world. The ancient world recognized this and believed that quartz was actually born of heavenly fire.[21] Meditating with these "stones of light" imbues the meditator with greater and greater light and life.

The Serpent of Fire

Always found on the fringe of optical imagery, the serpent plays an important role in linking the archetypes of quartz. As noted earlier, Asian motifs typically include sinewy, serpentine dragons clutching crystal balls. The image of fiery serpents and dragons bridges the crystal wand image and permeates the cultures of Mesoamerica, the Far East, and ancient Egypt.

Various cultures in Central and South America employ serpent motifs, often as coded symbols of deities ensconced in sacred spaces among the multitude of temples and pyramids. The luminous snake is occasionally depicted in quartz, such as the fire dragon and the serpent of light, found in the collection of the Seraphim Institute in Germany.[22] Since these cultures left behind sophisticated lapidary artifacts, it is likely they were able to annex celestial fire via crystal lenses and globes, too.

In other parts of the world, the serpent of fire was hidden in plain sight. In Egyptian mythology, the Uraeus was a solar serpent; its long body encircled a disc meant to be representative of the sun. Robert Temple suggests that this may actually be a stylized image of a crystal sun or lens, and the fiery serpent emanating from it is a distant relative of the cone of light descending from other crystal suns. The idea was preserved in Phoenician texts as a fiery serpent, which describes the process of finding the focal point of a lens or globe in order to set fire to what is beneath it.[23]

Aboriginal teachings of Australia include depictions of a creator god known as the Rainbow Serpent. In addition to the connection to the phallic nature of the wand, the serpent also draws a thread from the prism of the crystal wand to the lentoid optics of the crystal sun. The Rainbow Serpent, like the serpents of fire and light, emanates from crystals just as easily as it does from other sources.

The serpent often represents wisdom and regeneration. Just as the snake sheds its skin, the human soul sheds its body as it reincarnates. Crystals help us to attain perfection of embodiment by regenerating and revitalizing our entire beings. They fill us with light and they ignite our development. Crystals and shamans are close partners; as the serpent symbolizes wisdom permeating the temporal cycles of reincarnation, crystals are timeless teachers as well.

Clear Vision

No discussion of crystal balls and lenses would be complete without touching on crystal gazing. The art of scrying with rock crystal, either as a sphere or some other form, is frequently called "crystallomancy," and the outcome is attainment of clairvoyance, literally "clear vision." The art of scrying in crystal is analogous to using the obsidian mirror. While the effects are the same, the medium differs in that obsidian works to help the crystal-gazer face his or her shadows, whereas quartz requires one to stare at the brilliance and brightness of one's inner light.

The optical associations surrounding quartz throughout the ages are metaphors for en-*light*-enment. The journey through the crystal archetypes is pointed in the direction of becoming fully awakened. In truth, with self-actualization or enlightenment, the latent gifts and abilities of the mind are fully realized, too. With this comes clear seeing, not only in terms of peering into the past or the future, as seeing clearly is the result of the fully enlightened mind, ever focused on the eternal now.

Lenses magnify. They gather light. They correct for poor eyesight. In this manner, quartz crystal, for all its lenslike characteristics, also helps in correcting vision: it brings light to where there is darkness, and it magnifies whatever faint light is glowing within. When the crystal lens increases your light, everything in your life speeds up and awakens. For this reason, as the original purpose of the crystal spheres and lenses were forgotten, they nevertheless maintained their popularity into the Victorian era as ornamental talismans of good fortune. The delicate crystal balls, often set in silver, were thought by the Victorians to bring luck, healing, and protection; we can understand how this is the byproduct of quartz's mission, rather than its goal.

MEDITATION

THE CRYSTAL LIGHT

For this meditation a sphere of colorless, polished quartz is best. It does not have to be perfectly clear and free of inclusions, but a luminous quality is desirable. Avoid using "reconstituted" quartz spheres, as these are not actually quartz but glass, and they therefore lack the necessary crystalline structure needed. In the absence of such a stone in your toolbox, a tumbled or otherwise rounded stone will work well. Avoid using varieties of colored quartz, natural or otherwise, for this application.

The purpose of this meditation is twofold. First, it awakens your awareness of being an inseparable part of the source of all light in the universe. Second, it increases your personal light, which will result in relaxation, reduced negative mental patterns, and a greater sense of purpose. Before beginning, cleanse and clear the stone as needed. This exercise can also be adapted for use therapeutically on others; it is especially useful as a chakra therapy. Try using it briefly over each of the recipient's energy centers in order to clear and expand them.

As you commence the meditation, hold your quartz crystal in your dominant hand. As you breathe comfortably and consciously, allow your mind and body to relax fully. Raise the crystal above your head, holding it as high over your crown chakra as is comfortable. Visualize the stone collecting the light of the universe as you hold it aloft. This light may come from the sun, the moon, and the stars, as well as from Creator, from love, or from the earth. Picture this light descending from the sphere in a cone-shaped ray, and allow this light to reach a point directly on your crown chakra.

As you breathe, allow the light to flow into you on an inhalation. With every in-breath it floods you with more and more light, increasing the resonance of your being. As it permeates every particle of your body, let this light expand outward to fill your entire aura. When you feel saturated with light, you may send any excess back through the stone and out into the universe, or you can imagine it leaving your body through the soles of your feet and descending into Mother Earth.

QUARTZ AS AN ARCHETYPE: THE CRYSTALLINE SELF

In working with crystals, whether as wands or lenses or anything in-between, the goal is to unlock blocks to spiritual growth and healing. The primary functions of quartz are to empower the spiritual aspirant through the focusing, projective qualities of the wand, and to enlighten by magnifying and igniting with the lens. The structure, composition, and morphology of quartz contribute to its unique properties, both physical and spiritual, and they remind us that the most powerful tool for our growth is already with us.

Around the world, rock crystal has a mystical connection to the abode of spirits and gods alike. However, quartz is not an ethereal substance; it is a tangible and palpable mineral. It maintains a corporeal existence no matter how rarefied it is; this is the lesson of embodiment that quartz teaches. Crystals infuse our physical vehicles with light, which affects the innate crystallinity of our makeup.

The human body contains many crystalline and quasicrystalline compounds. Liquid crystals have been observed in our cells; DNA's repeating base pairs echo the periodic repetition that is pivotal to crystallinity itself. Apatite, a phosphate mineral, which naturally has a crystalline structure, can be found in bones and in teeth; and hemoglobin has more than one crystal form, contingent on whether it has bonded to oxygen. New Age thought presses the importance of becoming more crystalline as we undergo spiritual evolution, for our bodies must be ready to accept and flourish with new and higher frequencies.

Perhaps it is this call to becoming more crystalline that inspired shamans of yore to implant shards of quartz beneath the skin and to carve the likeness of the human form in quartz. Whenever an imbalance is experienced, either through illness or through negative mental or emotional patterns, the crystalline order is disrupted on one level or another. Crystals of all types, not just quartz, restore balance by repairing and restoring order. This may be geometric or chemical balance in the physical plane, or it may be a spiritual order that modifies thoughts or emotions to yield harmony. Crystals teach us to embody our inherent perfection, and quartz has been ubiquitously harnessed to demonstrate this lesson.

Crystal Skulls

Of all the topics related to the study of quartz, the mysteries of crystal skulls intrigue many of us the most. Skulls are often carved from a host of mineral and rock types, with quartz being the clear leader in popularity, both today and in ancient cultures. Many claims are made regarding these spiritual tools, and a detailed study of them merits its own book. In light of the scope of this book only quartz skulls will be examined, although virtually all skulls carved from minerals convey a common message.

The optical properties of crystal are among the traits most pertinent to its spiritual meanings. Several crystal skulls exhibit important and unusual applications of the optics of quartz, most notably the Mitchell-Hedges crystal skull, which has had its distinctive relationship with light appraised by scientists, artists, historians, and spiritual researchers alike. The skull is made from a block of clear quartz about the size of a small human cranium, measuring some 5 inches (13 cm) high, 7 inches (18 cm) long, and 5 inches wide. The lower jaw is detached. Crystallographer Frank Dorland conducted the most thorough study of this artifact. He determined that it was carved as a series of lenses and prisms that refract ambient light and focus it into the eyes and mouth of the skull.[24]

Other crystal skulls exhibit unusual optical effects, some of which are not comprehensible through the rational filter of science. For example, many skulls appear to change color and transparency as they are being worked with consciously. Among the sacred stones in my care is a crystal skull dating back to over a thousand years ago. Named for the district in Nepal from which he comes, "Mustang" weighs around six pounds and is fashioned from clear-to-milky Himalayan quartz. The skull has frequently demonstrated changes in his appearance, in which some portions go from opaque to perfectly clear, while others change from white to gold.

Crystal skulls are very nearly a worldwide phenomenon. They are reportedly found in the Americas, including Mexico, Guatemala, and Peru, with claims from the Diné (Navajo) that there is a crystal skull in their custodianship too. Skulls from Asia have been the most common discoveries in recent years, including those found in the Himalayas, in Tibet, Nepal, and presumably India, with even more coming from China and Mongolia. Crystal and stone heads can also be traced to Europe, such as a rose quartz skull from Russia, and examples carved from various rock types in Celtic lands. One skull, named "Compassion," is believed to have originated in Africa, although rumors of other African skulls have circulated for decades, and one named "Synergy" was found in Oceania.

There are many claims about the origins of crystal skulls, and many of these claims are conflicting. Most of the genuinely ancient skulls can be shown to exhibit tool marks, which is consistent with primitive tools and rudimentary lapidary technology, as should be expected of ancient artifacts. Quartz is a durable material, but it is eminently carvable with the right tools. Such carvings are the result of many hours of labor, a fact that points toward the sacred nature of these stones, as ancient cultures would only have attempted such a feat if they were motivated by more than aesthetic principles.

Some writers insist that crystal skulls are the result of long-lost cultures, extraterrestrial intervention, or spiritual phenomena; these ideas are further reinforced by the attitudes of mainstream academics, who consistently attempt to discredit the skulls as genuine artifacts. My own experience is that most genuinely old crystal skulls look and feel as though they were carved by more primitive tools. Even those with a high polish will exhibit telltale tool marks if examined under a high enough magnification. In my opinion, those which fail to display the appropriate surface markings are more than likely later fabrications.

The widespread distribution of crystal skulls points to one of the archetypal roles that quartz has assumed from culture to culture. The crystal skull represents the death of the ego and stripping away of the "surface" layer of life. Underneath this superficial glance there are commonalities that each person shares. The skull is quite literally a part of the body that we can't live without, thus it asks us to look toward our similarities as human beings, not our differences.

Crystal skulls also teach us to embrace the inevitable mortality that is part of life. Death and decay are natural. Our bodies will age, and when we die they will decompose and return to the earth. Since our faces are associated with our identity, and recognition of one another is usually by the face, the face of a fleshless skull depersonalizes death and makes it easier to embrace. Since the crystal skull is not made of organic tissue like our own skulls, it cannot decay. Quartz is not easily broken down in any environment on the surface of the earth. The message here is that there is a part of us that is impervious to the course of time; this same eternal part of ourselves exists beyond ego, fear, and illness. It is the divine spark within each person: the soul.

Crystal skulls, through their transparency and optical brilliance, teach us to become more crystalline at the core level. The skulls are important tools for learning to carry more light; they challenge us to embody it. It is impossible to do this in a state that is ruled by fear, so the death of the ego is a necessary precursor. If your ego lingers, combine obsidian with contemplation of the crystal skull, and it will fortify your efforts.

The skull is also the home of the brain, and the crystal skull therefore reminds us that the purpose of the brain, apart from organizing all the processes needed for life, is to be the portal to the higher mind. Crystal skulls carry an innate sense of wisdom and knowing. They have been regarded as recorders of the past and windows into the future. Tales about the knowledge contained within the crystal skulls abound, and these point to the idea that these skulls are programmed with information that will positively affect humanity in its quest for spiritual evolution. Each crystal skull that I have worked with has had its own distinct mission and personality, with some, such as the one in my collection, acting more as witnesses and guides rather than repositories of information.

Crystal skulls are the product of humankind's quest to better know itself; carving the likeness of a human skull out of quartz is part of the same drive for immortality that has resulted in grandiose tombs and exquisite funerary goods. The skulls are elegant reminders that this immortality and self-knowledge is already within each of us. Although our physical bodies will not last forever, the true self never dies. By connecting to this verity in a visceral way, we can crystallize our whole being and fully embrace and embody the light of the soul.

The Crystal Heart

Whereas the crystal skull helps the psyche detach from the ego to allow light through to the physical embodiment, the crystal heart clears the passage for crystallinity to manifest at the emotional level. Heart-shaped gemstone amulets can be traced back to ancient Egypt, where they were called *ab*.[25] While carnelian, jasper, and lapis lazuli were popular choices in the ancient world, hearts carved of other mediums, including quartz, are not unknown. One example discovered in Mesoamerica is touted as having been created in Atlantis.[26] The use of crystal hearts was common in Europe, and the practice culminated in ornate examples of crystal hearts, sometimes adorned with precious gemstones, such as one fashioned by Fabergé.[27]

When a sufficient amount of light has been anchored in our beings, the emotional body can no longer house conflicting or antagonistic emotional patterns. Our belief systems, which inform our behavior and feelings, are gently rewired in order to promote a cohesive mental-emotional platform for spiritual evolution. The heart has always held a sacred place in spiritual traditions. Modern science indicates that it is much more important than previously believed. It generates electrical and magnetic fields much greater than those of the brain, which indicates that it may be an important sensory organ. The heart is also viewed as the bridge between the upper and lower energy centers of the body; it is literally at the core of our being.

The crystal heart represents emotional enlightenment. This stage in our evolution is born out of compassion, wisdom, and love. The ego knows only conditional love. The crystal skull shows us the path to egolessness; the natural progression, to the crystal heart, generates unconditional love.

The crystal heart comes full circle from the mirror of the heart that is obsidian, touched on in the first chapter. Obsidian is a smoking mirror, and it teaches the spiritual aspirant to gently polish the heart in order to reflect perfection outward. Obsidian, however, reflects our shadow side before accomplishing anything else. With the crystal heart there is no smoke between the mirrors; there is only light. When you realize the crystal heart, others see that you have found the God-self within, and it inspires them to do likewise. The beauty of the crystal heart is that it reflects the luminous nature of the soul to others; you allow others to see their own divinity and perfection in your heart. This, in turn, illumines and crystallizes their hearts so that they may pay it forward and continue the momentum.

The Crystalline Body

Our physical incarnation is the product of the organizational forces of the soul, the mind, and the subtle bodies. The physical body responds to environmental stimuli, the foods we eat, the thoughts we think, and the people we meet. Countless recent studies have shown that science is beginning to comprehend how powerful techniques such as meditation, qigong, Reiki, yoga, and other modalities may be in effecting change at the physical level. There may soon be controlled, tangible proof of the benefit of gemstones on our well-being, too.

The human body shares certain traits with the mineral kingdom, at least in terms of its crystalline components. Our physical makeup includes a matrix of both liquid and solid crystals and quasicrystals. Chief among these are constituents of blood, the mineral salts of our cells, elements of bone, proteins, and, of course, DNA. Each of these compounds of which our physical manifestation is comprised exhibits degrees of coherence that mirror the crystalline state such as that found in quartz.

Of all of these crystalline components, it is the genetic constitution of the body that displays the most similarities to quartz. As quartz forms, it adds on new silica bases in the form of tetrahedral units of silicon and oxygen in a helical pattern. Similarly, our DNA is a sequence of bases arranged helically. The geometric arrangement of DNA places it in communication with the higher levels of consciousness; it can be said that our genetic makeup "is but one step-down transformation if a vast network of interconnected Life-codes. The pattern and content of the physical DNA originates on the level of the Higher Self."[28] Much like quartz, DNA is also hexagonal in its morphology.[29]

The spiral form of DNA also follows the rotation of polarized light traveling through quartz crystal. As light enters a clear piece of quartz, the wave patterns organize themselves into an optimal level of coherence in the polarized state. When it travels parallel to the central axis of the crystal, it is further influenced by the crystal in that it rotates, forming a helical wave pattern as it journeys through the crystal. This helix of light actually results in a state of entanglement, wherein two photons, or particle waves of light energy, become interdependent at the quantum level. Any action influencing one photon will have an identical impact on its entangled "twin."

DNA shares this spiral form, and like quartz it also has an intimate relationship with light. Quartz crystals exhibit piezoelectricity in that when the crystal lattice is mechanically deformed in one way or another (by striking, squeezing, or otherwise applying force), the crystals will emit an electrical charge. Similarly, applying electrical energy will cause the crystal to oscillate. One of the side effects of this is a property called "triboluminescence," which allows photons to be emitted as the quartz generates electrons due to piezoelectricity. All of this is merely quartz's response to the mechanical stress in an effort to maintain balance.

The DNA in each cell of our bodies also emits light. This means that both quartz and DNA are hexagonal crystals capable of emitting light under the correct circumstances.[30] The laws of sympathetic resonance suggest that each would vibrate in harmony with the other, thus when you connect with quartz and its archetypes you activate the crystalline potential encoded within every cell of your body; this in turn awakens your spiritual potential and moves your whole being toward a more evolved, crystalline state.

The undulating helix of DNA may also connect to the optical attributes of quartz in an unexpected way. Anthropological research has found connections between the legend of the "cosmic serpent" and DNA among native cultures.[31] The serpentine form of DNA resembles the serpents of fire, light, and rainbow discussed earlier in this chapter. Quartz crystals awaken the inner wisdom of the body by vibrating in sympathy to the cosmic serpent of DNA itself. Since quartz conveys a message primarily connected to light, both spiritual and literal, connecting to the archetype of the crystalline body kindles a lightening of our physical vehicle at the core level.

Research suggests that it is possible to raise our level of crystallinity. Through spiritual practices and by connecting to the mineral kingdom, "we may actually be able to *increase* the degree of our internal coherence, or liquid crystallinity."[32] This equates to greater organization on all levels of manifestation, although it is most visible at the microscopic level. Greater coherence of our liquid crystalline matrix will in turn affect the resonant frequency of the body, which functions like an antenna for our electromagnetic presence.

The body is a transducer of mental, spiritual, and emotional forces. Much in the way that quartz converts physical input into electrical and photonic output, and vice versa, through piezoelectricity the human body interprets and responds to the stimuli provided by the subtle bodies. The body is a sophisticated biological transmitter-receiver attuned to the mind, heart, and spirit. When the systems of the body achieve greater coherence, they may be able to refine and amplify their roles in translating and radiating the signals from higher levels of organization.

Most spiritual traditions discuss some sort of body of light, usually taught after the person has attained a major milestone in spiritual growth. This light body is meant to represent our spiritually perfected state completely integrated into our physical embodiment. Quartz helps us move toward this idealized form through its message of embodiment. Connecting to the archetype of the crystalline self can increase the integrity and coherence of the body's physical tissues, which allow them to anchor more and more light. Quartz prepares us on all levels for the next stage in our evolution and spiritual development.

MEDITATION

CRYSTALLIZING ONESELF

For this meditation, choose any piece of quartz that calls to you. It can be polished or natural, clear or cloudy. Cleanse the crystal and hold it in whichever hand feels most comfortable for meditation.

Begin by breathing consciously and slowly. Allow each breath to relax the body and mind further and further. As you become more relaxed, shift your attention to the crystal. Imagine that with each in-breath the crystal's light moves through your hand, up your arm, and courses through your body. As you exhale, you release any patterns of disharmony or noncrystalline frequencies from your being. Each in-breath increases the crystalline energy circulating through you.

After several minutes, hold the crystal to your heart center. Visualize your breath entering through the heart, filtered through the piece of quartz against your chest. The breath is luminous and dazzling. Let the breath accumulate in the heart; each inhalation allows your heart to become more and more crystalline, until it is radiant like a gemstone.

When your heart has achieved a crystalline brilliance, turn the focus outward. Expand the light outward, filling the room. Inhale more light, and as you exhale gently push the perimeter of light to encircle a greater and greater radius. Gradually, this light encircles the globe. Everything that it touches begins to crystallize and radiate light. Intend that your luminous meditation will serve all living beings and Earth herself.

When you feel ready, gradually withdraw your attention from the planet as a whole and return to an awareness of yourself in meditation. Gently focus on the breath. Send any excess energy into the earth beneath you. When you feel grounded and secure, open your eyes.

QUARTZ IN CRYSTAL HEALING

More than any other type of mineral or rock known to crystal therapists, quartz crystals and their many cousins are indispensable and universal tools. Many of the most popular healing stones in the toolboxes of twenty-first-century shamans and gemstone therapists are classified as varietals of quartz. In the context of this chapter the healing properties of quartz will be discussed as pertaining to transparent and translucent colorless quartz, as well as generically applying to all members of the crystalline categories of quartz, including clear quartz, amethyst, smoky quartz, citrine, etc.

Easily applied at all levels of manifestation, quartz is a genuine, all-purpose healing tool. It is versatile, and it may be applied as natural crystal points or as faceted stones, as wands and tumbled stones, or as any other type of form. The primary function of quartz is to promote multidimensional balance, bringing body, mind, and spirit into perfect harmony. In modern applications of gemstone therapy, quartz is the first tool with which students become acquainted, because its many uses outnumber other stones. It is taught that quartz enhances vitality by attracting *chi*, or the life force; it also attracts a full complement of the seven color rays, thus restoring all systems to equilibrium at a gradual tempo.[33]

Working with quartz to effect therapeutic transformation can be directed through intent, thus allowing the practitioner to focus on a desired outcome. Quartz can be applied to the aura of the recipient, placed on the body on its own or as an amplifier for other gems. It can be used as a meditative spotlight, centering the attention on achieving the necessary result. Quartz tools are highly customizable for co-creation by programming specific intentions, which greatly enhances the healing process.

EXERCISE

PROGRAMMING A CRYSTAL

The following methodology has been adapted from several sources, although the main inspiration comes from the Vogel programming technique. Marcel Vogel was at one time an IBM research scientist who later turned toward an exploration of psychic phenomena and crystal healing. His teachings and techniques have left an indelible mark on the spiritual community, and his methods are reliable and easy to master. Although this technique is presented here in the chapter on quartz, any stone can be imbued with a specific program using this procedure. The first breath is aimed at cleansing your crystal, effectively wiping the slate clean for whichever intention you would like to co-create.

Select the crystal with which you would like to work. Clear your mind and center yourself in gratitude before beginning. Holding the stone comfortably cradled in your hands, begin to visualize white light filling your body with every breath. With each successive breath, the light inundates your being, dissolving any blockages or disharmonious frequencies. When you sense that you are saturated with this energy, breathe in deeply and exhale sharply and rapidly through the nose into the stone.

Next, focus on your intention. It can be a simple concept, such as love or healing, or you can choose a more involved message. Try to choose a word or phrase that most simply describes the outcome. Visualize the end result or any symbol representative thereof. Again, breathe this energy into your body; allow it to permeate every nook and cranny of your being. When you have reached saturation, fill your lungs completely and exhale sharply through the nostrils as before, directly into the crystal. Afterward, bring the stone to your heart and offer gratitude in order to complete the process.

More than one intention can be combined in a single piece of quartz; however, if you do this, the programs chosen should be harmonious. Marcel always used the following combination: peace, well-being, and love.

As a tool for healing at the physical level, quartz is often the first and only stone needed. Applying quartz infuses a target area with life force, which promotes healthy circulation of energy and expedites the healing process. This mechanism can eliminate energetic blockages, disrupt the signals stemming from mental and emotional causes of illness, and focus the awareness on the underlying patterns of disease in order to release them.

Quartz is especially helpful for pain management; placing quartz directly on an injured area can reduce not only pain but also inflammation, redness, stiffness, and signs of infection. Quartz may accelerate the repair of damaged tissues as well as target pathogens in order to help the immune system locate pockets of infection. Typically, polished and tumbled specimens of quartz are excellent tools for any of these applications.

Using terminated crystals can also direct healing energies into physical areas. Point them at a target zone to infuse it with energy, or reverse the direction of the crystal to help siphon off the unwanted or disharmonious vibrations. Alternately, a crystal can be held in the receptive hand while the other hand is placed on the area in need of healing.

Quartz is especially suited to healing the lungs. The inherent clarity and coolness of quartz is often connected to the element of air, making it an excellent vitalizing stone for the respiratory system in a therapeutic context. Placing quartz on the chest or wearing a strand of quartz beads is an efficient way to direct quartz's focus onto the lungs. High-altitude quartz such as crystals from the Himalayas also makes an exemplary healing tool for the respiratory system; it brings a refreshing energy, not unlike the unadulterated air of faraway high mountains.

More important than its characteristics of physical healing, rock crystal makes an excellent tool for healing the mind and the emotions. The archetypes of quartz promote directionality and focus. These translate to follow-through and concentration when applied in healing. Natural and polished crystals of quartz are wandlike in appearance, and they empower the mind to take responsibility for the conditions around it. This can also result in more intentional manifestation, wherein quartz appears to magnify the results of the co-creative process; in reality, quartz is cohering the mental and emotional frequencies of the person such that they work together, unilaterally effecting the same transformation.

Quartz, for all its optical imagery, cannot escape the principles of insight and clarity on the mental emotional levels. Quartz can engender stillness and silence in the mind, which supports meditative states and helps neutralize the background "noise" in one's mind. This silencing of subsidiary thoughts grants peace, tranquility, and clarity to anyone conscientiously working with quartz. As a result, patterns of mental and emotional disease can be gently erased. In this manner, quartz is efficacious in clearing patterns of worry, anger, depression, and anxiety. As it calms the mind, quartz sympathetically cools the hot emotions and warms the cold, dispassionate ones. Quartz crystal is a poor thermal conductor and is easily distinguished from lookalikes because it is generally cool to the touch. This feature of quartz can be used to similarly cool down anger, rage, confusion, and paranoia. Conversely, because the optics of crystal allow it to condense light enough to ignite heat and fire, quartz's healing energies can be directed toward lethargic, stagnant mental patterns or used for warming bitter, worrisome, detached, mournful, and frigid dispositions.

The traditional lunar associations of quartz imbue it with all the energetic qualities of the moon. This being the case, it is the quintessential gemstone for providing balance of emotions, gaining insight into temporal cycles, and conceptualizing the ebb and flow of life. Quartz is capable of transforming or transducing energies, thus allowing one to bridge the physical with the mental, and the mental with the spiritual planes. Quartz allows its user to recognize the interdependency of all dimensions.

Spiritually, quartz is a stone of mastery. While it is the most basic of healing stones, it is also the most adept. The myriad forms in which it is continually being discovered account for the diverse and ever-evolving nature of this crystal's healing powers. Because it apparently amplifies our intentions and our efforts, rock crystal is a potent adjunct to any spiritual practice. It offers clarity and illumination on the spiritual path and can assist you in achieving self-discipline.

Varieties of Quartz

There are more varieties of quartz known to mineral collectors than probably any other crystal. For this reason, only a few are discussed here. The members of the quartz clan listed below have been chosen for their relevance to the archetypes above, as well as for their therapeutic value.

Cathedral Lightbrary Crystals

In the previous chapter, the structure of these brilliant crystals was described as resembling the spires of a Gothic cathedral. Cathedral lightbraries are most commonly found in Brazil, where they may be clear, smoky, or citrine quartz, although varieties can be found worldwide in many other types of quartz, too.

Of all the forms of quartz, these may be my favorite configurations. To recognize a true cathedral, there should be a luminous quality within the stone. These crystals are seemingly alive for their inner light. The cathedrals, as mentioned in the previous chapter, are a representation of the synthesis of both study and practice. They connect the mental and spiritual bodies to foster greater spiritual growth. The lightbraries are also superb crystals for connecting to cosmic intelligence. They are akin to record keeper crystals (or trigonic crystals, discussed later in this chapter) in that they are often repositories of information. However, in meditation one often finds that these crystals vibrate on a galactic level. They can make the impersonal wisdom of the stars more attainable and tangible to the human consciousness.

Cathedral crystals are excellent stones to use in sacred space because they anchor the harmony of the spheres into your personal sanctuary. Cathedral lightbraries offer guidance and support on the spiritual path, and they are best met in meditation. They can be held or contemplated in a meditative state; after attaining resonance with them, try visualizing your consciousness or light body entering the stone and exploring the rooms within.

Crystal Skulls

Crystal skulls of any variety of mineral are powerful accelerators in the healing process. Their archetypal role has been discussed previously, but they also offer therapeutic benefits. Crystal skulls help us to embrace the power of the mind. Your skull is the keeper of your brain, which on the physical plane connects to your mind; the crystal skull is a symbol of the power of the mind for illuminating and crystallizing your reality. Working with this tool can soothe the mind as well as intensify the focus of the mind during meditation and healing work.

A crystal skull, given the relationship of crystal skulls worldwide, is a visual representation of mortality. While crystal skulls are sometimes regarded as macabre illustrations of the inevitability of death, the skull, too, inspires hope as it challenges you to live each day fully, as if it could be your last. Crystal skulls show that with endings there come new beginnings. They are the alpha and the omega, manifest in a single carving. This energetic resonance implies that the skulls are valuable tools for initiating change, entering new cycles, and for opening the inner vision to new vistas.

Himalayan Quartz

Himalayan quartz describes high-altitude crystals from a variety of mining sites throughout the Himalayas, in Asia. These crystals may come from Tibet, Nepal, India, or Pakistan. Although their appearance differs greatly from one location to another, each of the varieties shares certain common traits. Several crystal skulls are carved from Himalayan quartz; they feature in certain tantric rituals of Himalayan mystics.

Himalayan quartz emphasizes stillness. The mountain range is the highest in the world, with many mountains sacred to the spiritual traditions found in that region. Holding a piece of quartz from the Himalayas can impart an air of holiness. These stones are often strikingly clear, and the inclusions in many of them only add to their beauty. Himalayan quartz promotes a relationship with forms of Asian spirituality; it can help us bridge cultures and anchor the high and pure vibrations of the Himalayan mountains. They enhance meditation, healing, fasting, and channeling.[34]

A type of Himalayan quartz called Tibetan black quartz—also called "black phantom quartz" or "black spot quartz"—refers to clear, double-terminated quartz crystals from Tibet that exhibit various dark inclusions. Many of these crystals contain enhydros inclusions, in which water and gas bubbles are trapped during the crystal's formation. These are dynamic healing tools because their double-terminated form allows for a clear channel of energy, while the iron and carbon inclusions anchor the high frequencies carried by Tibetan crystals. These stones can be used to clear blocked energy centers and to achieve balance.

Nepalese alpine crystals go by different names depending on their exact source and distributor. Mostly available from Ganesh Himal and Kangchenjunga, these crystals exhibit strange morphologies. Many are included with chlorite and actinolite and have graceful, elongated prism faces. Occasionally, crystals with growth interference from other minerals, generally calcite, can also be found. These crystals sometimes resemble the mountains from which they come. Nepalese quartz tends to be mined by hand with tremendous care.

These crystals awaken a sense of custodianship for the earth, and they are deeply compassionate. The addition of chlorite to their makeup grants an amplified healing quality, and they are wonderful tools for any crystal therapist.

Nirvana quartz is a type of Himalayan crystal found in the Kullu Pass of Northern India. These crystals were first made available several years ago when miners discovered them beneath receding glaciers. Their complex morphologies resemble the icy glaciers where they were found, and they frequently exhibit unusual angles and etchings; many are also trigonic crystals. They can be both clear and pinkish, not unlike Lemurian seed crystals, discussed below. The surprising geometries in which they are found are the result of growth interference, in which the quartz formed alongside calcite, or possibly other minerals, which later dissolved and left only their impressions on the faces of the quartz crystals.

Nirvana quartz is an evolutionary stone. It imparts the typical sensation of stillness often associated with Himalayan crystals, and in this silence there is an infusion of peace and trust. I find these crystals to awaken faith in the process of planetary evolution that we are currently undergoing. They were discovered only as glaciers receded, apparently a product of global climate change.

Mother Earth, in all her infinite wisdom, has had these crystals waiting in repose for the right time to release them, and the mechanism for their revelation is generally a cause for great concern because of the environmental impact of climate change. It is as if the Earth Mother has sent these crystals to help us cope with the evolution of ourselves and our planet. They seem to convey the message that "it's okay that things are changing" because they are meant to shift. Nirvana crystals help one to embrace destiny, and they can also spur action to change for the better. They awaken a sense of responsibility and stewardship while facilitating a deep communion with the intelligence of the heart center.[35]

Laser Wands

Laser wands are characterized by a long, tapering morphology. They often have bent or uneven prism faces and small terminal facets. The shape of these crystals allows energy moving through them to travel quickly, ultimately being compressed into a tight beam as it exits the point of the crystal. The laser wands are not always the most conventionally beautiful crystals, but they are the power tools of the crystal toolbox. Katrina Raphaell first described these crystals in her book *Crystal Healing.*[36]

Laser wand crystals exemplify focus and discipline. Because the energy that flows through them is such a compact beam, it helps to narrow one's mental focus to a similar focal point. Meditating with them cultivates discipline and perseverance. Many of them feel very ancient and wise; indeed, they may have been seeded by ancient intelligences to carry their teachings into the current moment.

As healing tools, laser wands are indispensable. They can be used to excise negative thought forms, cut cords, detach entities, and break down blockages. Use them with care, for their energy can be invasive, like a scalpel. Cut only what is necessary when performing any sort of psychic surgery. Afterward, anchor the changes created by sealing the area with the soft, nurturing energies of a stone such as rose quartz, aventurine, or quartzite.

An alternative method to cutting out pieces of the energy anatomy is to harness the power of the laser wand through meditative focus. When a mental or emotional pattern is cut out of the subtle body, there is a high chance that its root cause remains, which will encourage the discordant energy to return. Instead, meditating with the laser wand can point toward this root cause. When the feeling or belief that is the source of the discordant energy has been located, visualize the tight, laserlike energy of the wand penetrating and encapsulating it. When it has been saturated with the light carried by the crystal, it can be broken down and removed with ease. Not only are the results more likely permanent, the energetic anatomy of the client does not undergo any sort of surgical trauma.

Lemurian Seed Crystals

Lemurian seed crystals (LSCs for short) were the very first formations of quartz that initiated any sort of metaphysical experience on my personal journey. They appear to be a specialized form of laser wand (see above) and were first made available at the end of the last millennium. These crystals originate from a mine in Serra do Cabral, located in Minas Gerais, Brazil. They display a Muzo habit, which results in a triangular, or nearly triangular, appearance of the crystal at the termination when viewed in cross-section. This results from an environment that favors the growth of three of the prism faces, thus crowding out the other three such that they gradually taper to nothing. Nearly all of the LSCs have a matte finish, with horizontal striations along the wider three prism faces.

The overall shape of these crystals is reminiscent of laser wands. In fact, the majority of the LSCs function as very specialized forms of these tools. In therapeutic applications, they may be substituted perfectly. Apart from this aspect, the LSCs make intimate tools for meditation and spiritual growth. They have an exceedingly gentle presence as well as an innate wisdom. It has been posited that the growth lines along the prism faces represent records of information seeded by the Lemurian consciousness. Meditating with the striations held against the heart or the third eye is an easy way to integrate their teachings.

Lemurian seed crystals preach a message of unity to all humankind. In this regard they tap into the collective field created by the LSCs as they spread around the globe. Each person who is co-creating with them, whether consciously or not, has helped to create a web of light around the globe; each point on this grid is one of the LSCs. The mission that they are enacting is to unify the people of Earth toward love and compassion, as well as to reclaim the spiritual birthright and abilities said to have been used freely on the lost continent of Lemuria. These crystals are very heart-centered, and they can help one tap into one's spiritual gifts.

Although the original Lemurian crystals are from Brazil, specimens meeting the morphological requirements have been found in several other locations. Oftentimes they may be formed as entire deposits, while in other instances they may be strewn among crystals of more typical growth habits. Examples of LSCs can be found in Colombia, Arkansas, Australia, Russia, Mozambique, China, Zambia, and Mexico. While generally comprised of very clear quartz, they sometimes occur with mineral deposits at or near the surface, rendering the stones a brown, red, green, orange, pink, or yellow color. Rarely, they may also occur in smoky and amethystine forms of quartz.

Himalayan Lemurians are a new find of LSCs, first made available in 2015. They come from a high-altitude pocket of quartz among the Himalayas. They have a bucolic, tingling presence when held, and they represent stillness and serenity. There is an air of innocence in these crystals, perhaps due to the newness of their arrival. These crystals have a joyous, playful presence, which helps one to live more presently and contentedly.

Mozambique Lemurians are also called "soul shepherds." Similar to their Lemurian cousins in Brazil and the Himalayas, they are characterized by horizontal lineations on the surfaces of the prism faces. They too display the familiar matte texture on the surface, although they are generally not as finely tapered as other LSCs. Most of the crystals arrive broken and beaten, and that is part of their charm. In addition to other properties associated with LSCs, the Mozambican crystals guide our souls toward their highest expressions. They are potent stones, spiritual power tools that are excellent for shamanic applications of healing and soul retrieval. Many of them have tinges of gold from superficial traces of iron oxide, which strengthens and aligns their focus toward the light.

Moon Quartz

Although it rarely forms euhedral crystal points, moon quartz is easily recognized for its unique appearance and optics. Moon quartz is named for its hazy, silvery gray contraluz, an appearance of being lit from within. The effect is generally caused by minute inclusions in the form of needlelike or tubular structures that softly diffuse light passing through the stone, with a decidedly lunar glow. Similar stones are also occasionally called "transformation quartz" and "girasol," and these may sometimes be tinged with other colors, such as lilac, lavender, and rose.

Moon quartz is a soft, gentle member of the quartz family that assists in making changes; it subtly helps new patterns take root as their energetic counterparts propagate in our auras. The mystical contraluz effect of this stone encourages a diffuse, relaxing energy, almost like a fine mist, infusing the aura with whichever goal or intention is focused into the stone. As this frequency saturates the aura, it begins to manifest elsewhere in our lives, too.

There is a gentle femininity to this stone, and the lunar connection makes for an ideal tool to assist with intuition and connection to motherly archetypes. Moon quartz is typically crisscrossed with a network of fine tubes or needles, which represent the energetic matrix and the communication networks within it. Wearing or gazing into this stone puts one in touch with this communication system, thereby increasing receptivity to intuitive information.

Phantom Crystals

When growth conditions are just right, quartz crystals may contain a spectral outline of a crystal frozen within its core. This shadowy inclusion is referred to as a "phantom," and it occurs when changes in the growth conditions encourage pauses during the crystal's formation. When the crystal slows or stops its growth, other substances may be included around the surface before resuming. This action delineates a shadowy, insubstantial snapshot of what the crystal once looked like when it was younger. Oftentimes phantoms occur in many phases of growth, and the pattern is repeated through the stone.

Phantom crystals help to pierce the veil of time and memory, which enables them to assist with past-life recall and with healing traumatic memories from this or any lifetime. Phantom crystals are connected to liminal zones; the appearance of the phantom resembles a boundary or line of demarcation between the inner and outer territories. Because of this quality, crystals with phantoms facilitate the crossing of barriers during spiritual development. They can provide access to nonphysical planes, including the Akashic records, as well as assist in contacting your guides or teachers. Phantom crystals also incorporate the energy of whichever mineral or combination of minerals comprises the phantoms.

The inner phantom appears to be a crystal within a crystal. Meditating with these stones can help in integrating the archetype of the crystalline self because they represent the axiom that we are already innately perfect; it is only necessary to see this latent perfection in order to actualize it. In so doing, the phantom crystal can also yield unexpected results with other spiritual pursuits by unlocking our spiritual gifts, such as clairvoyance, clairaudience, astral projection, or lucid dreaming.

Rutilated Quartz

Under the right conditions, as quartz crystallizes it can enclose fine, needlelike crystals of rutile, an oxide of titanium. These crystals can resemble metallic arrows or fibers within the host quartz, and they are sometimes accompanied by crystals of hematite. Rutilated quartz has been known as *fleches d'amour,* or "arrows of love," and as "Venus's hair" because of the appearance of rutile.

Rutilated quartz combines the light-related imagery of quartz with the fibers or needles of rutile. The rutile can serve as a metaphorical path for energy such as light to follow. Rutilated quartz serves as a means for enhancing communication and for amplification of any message in light of this. Rutile, because of its titanium content, also has a strengthening effect. It can be very penetrative, helping you focus on energetic blockages and working to erode them. The presence of titanium can lend a sense of self-discipline, thus making rutilated quartz an important auxiliary tool during the development of any new skill or application thereof.

The traditional association with images of Cupid's arrows and

Aphrodite's hair also lends this crystal to the work of co-creation on an emotional level. It can provide a straightforward outlet when communicating one's emotions, and it helps to guide messages directly to the heart of the receiver. This helps the speaker find clarity and ease of expression, and helps the listener hear the truth of the message without personal bias.

Scepter Crystals

Occasionally, minerals will display a second stage of crystal growth that caps or crowns the original body of the crystal. This type of growth habit is called a "scepter," as it resembles a wand or staff with a ceremonial point. Scepterlike growth is often responsible for types of complex growth in quartz, including elestial crystals. Scepters may occur in any variety of quartz, occasionally even as combinations, such as a smoky cap on white quartz.

Scepter crystals convey power and authority to those who carry them. They are tools for learning to become the ruler of your own destiny. As energy is directed through a scepter, a sense of weight and fortitude is added before exiting. This yields a more powerful punch than your average quartz crystal.

Scepters are powerful adjuncts to other healing stones. They work like a honing device; when the cause for a condition or scenario is unknown, try adding a scepter crystal to the stones already in use. The scepter directs the energies into the heart of the target, whether it is a confusing physical condition or a tangled mass of mental patterns. Scepters penetrate the symptoms without being misled by them. Instead, these crystals always point toward the root of any situation.

Scepter crystals can also resolve problems related to masculinity, by way of sympathetic resonance. Their overtly phallic form can tap into the primal essence of maleness, which can be used to release issues connected to it. Scepters can also add balance to the feminine polarity without overpowering it.

Trigonic Quartz

Trigonic formations are triangular marks that typically occur on the termination faces of some crystals. When raised slightly and pointed upward, these are traditionally called "record keepers," a term coined by crystal healing pioneer Katrina Raphaell. However, when found as downward-pointing triangles etched or incised into the face, these are the true trigonic crystals.

Trigonic quartz works at the blueprint level for healing. Not unlike the energy of the diamond, which also frequently manifests with trigonic etchings, this formation of quartz seeks to heal and upgrade the patterning that makes up the fabric of our existence. They are visionary crystals that put us in direct communication with our superconsciousness. Connecting with these crystals is profound. They are stones for soul-level healing and awareness.[37] The triangles etched into them resemble the geometric pattern of our light bodies, and they can push our consciousness out into the realm of shamanic journeying in order to comprehend the blueprints that we carry.

The trigonics are multidimensional tools; they facilitate contact with the oversoul. This provides insight into the patterns that we have at the personal level; such awareness is often all it takes to release and heal these beliefs and emotions. Trigonic quartz is an initiatory stone; the energy contained in this crystal formation imparts movement to the soul. Co-creating with these crystals can be life-changing; use them only after personal spiritual preparation, and be ready for the shift to occur!

Related Stones

Opal

Opal is a relative of quartz. It forms as cryptocrystalline spheres of silica in lieu of the rigorous tetrahedral lattice for which quartz is so well known. Opals contain up to 21 percent water, and the distribution of this water, in conjunction with the uniformity of the size of the silica spheres, is responsible for the clarity and opalescent brilliance, or inner fire, of precious opals. These amorphous gemstones can be found in a variety of colors, from the reds, oranges, browns, and yellows of the jellylike fire opals, to the whites, blues, and blacks of precious opals. Massive semitranslucent or opaque stones are available in colors such as white, gray, brown, green, pink, and purple, from a number of locations worldwide. Hyaline opals are water-clear, and they can typically be found as thin crusts or films over other mineral formations.

Opal shares equal merit with quartz as being an all-purpose stone. The notion dates back some time, and it stems from the idea that fine opals exhibit the benefits of all gemstones because they bear the full spectrum of colors.

Quartzite

Quartzite can actually refer to two formations. The first is a metamorphic rock descended from sandstone that has undergone changes due to the pressure and heat from the birth of mountains. The tiny grains of quartz sand have been compressed and cemented together to form a tough rock. The second material is usually a massive, nontransparent form of quartz; it is sometimes referred to as "milky quartz."

Quartzite of either classification is a gently stabilizing stone. It is slow-acting, like the formation of mountains, but it can help to direct and anchor the changes we are experiencing. It can be used as a tool to remember to slow down and breathe, as well as for delicately instilling a peaceful sense of stillness. Wearing quartzite is sometimes contraindicated when combined with other stones or when worn for long periods of time, but as a therapeutic tool it can assist in assimilating and maintaining the positive transitions initiated by other gemstones.[38] Raw pieces of quartzite, easily found in nature, are easy tools for supporting the benefits of other gemstones. Use them in pairs placed beside other stones during a laying-on-of-stones to slow the action of brisk, erratic changes, or place a piece of quartzite on a target area after completing a treatment with other stones to deepen the benefits and ensure longlasting changes.

Because it lacks the optical clarity of crystalline quartz, quartzite can be used by those who are resistant to integrating the lessons of quartz's archetypes. It helps to begin a gradual transition toward acceptance and comprehension of the mission of quartz without feeling overwhelming. In cases where someone is hypersensitive to crystal energy, work up to high-power crystals by first using softening, counterbalancing quartzite. Metamorphic quartzite, which is essentially a rarefied and reincarnated sandstone, can additionally be used to help manifest goals by cementing together the separate pieces of our dreams.

7

DIAMOND

The Unconquerable and the Thunderbolt

More than any other gemstone, the diamond has earned its place as a precious stone that beguiles nearly everyone. This crystalline gem is prized for its relative rarity, brilliance, and durability, all of which outshine most other minerals on Earth. As a tool for spiritual growth, diamonds have been held in high regard in many cultures throughout history, as this stone holds the key to unlocking our highest potential.

Diamond is a mineral substance that forms from a fairly common element: it is pure carbon, a true native element. It is generally presumed that diamonds are birthed deep within the earth and are brought to the surface by vertical structures (pipes) of kimberlite and related rocks. Although the most sought-after diamonds are those of gem quality and famously colorless, diamonds range in quality, color, and clarity, from transparent shades of clear to white, yellow, golden and brown, blue, green, orange, pink, and red to the more opaque varieties with metallic lusters. Black, silver, and grey diamonds are common compared to the gem standard of the ideal, colorless stone.

Diamonds are classified in the cubic crystal system. They grow in a multitude of forms, with cubic, dodecahedral, octahedral, and related shapes being the most frequently occurring. Classically, the octahedron is the most recognizable crystal form. It contributes to the optical brilliance and even the characteristic hardness of this stone.

While diamonds were certainly known among some ancient cultures, their high hardness precludes them from ever having been faceted until more recently in the history of lapidary arts. Diamonds are considered to be the hardest known natural substance, ranking with a coefficient of 10 on the Mohs scale of hardness of 1 to 10. The diamond is many times more resistant to scratching than even the second-hardest stone, corundum. The compact, covalent bonds among the carbon atoms that comprise the diamond are responsible for the hardness, and they also account for several other interesting properties. Diamond's tightly packed carbon atoms help it to achieve a higher-than-average density, despite the intrinsic lightness of carbon itself. And it is this density that accounts for diamond's high refractive index: as light passes through more electrons in a given substance, it is slowed down more and more; this means that in the structure of diamond crystals "the electrons are packed together very densely and are tightly bound in the structure, so the velocity of light is reduced."[1]

Despite ancient beliefs that diamonds are impervious to heat and can affect magnetism, these gemstones are excellent conductors of heat. They are four times more effective than copper in this application, and they can burn at a high enough temperature.[2] Unlike more plentiful types of carbon, such as graphite or the plethora of carbonate minerals, diamonds are formed only under the most intense heat and pressure, sometimes within stars. And combustible though it may be, the diamond is able to survive many extremes.

In history, the telltale hardness of diamond is responsible for its name. The word *diamond* can be traced back to the Greek expression *adamas,* which means "not conquered" or "not tamed." While throughout history many stones were conflated with diamonds, to ancient people *adamant* referred to a substance that could overcome any other. As the word traveled through languages on its path to modern renderings, it was occasionally called *dieu amant* in Middle French, meaning "god lover," a close approximation of the Greek root word, referring to the stone's divine connection. This yielded the modern French word *diamant*.

To the ancient Hebrews, both *yahalom* and *shamir* are applied to diamond; the first word means "stone of great brilliance and value," while the second is translated as "something very hard."[3] In biblical passages these are sometimes merely rendered as *adamant,* a stone surpassing the hardness of all others. Because it is probable that true diamonds were relatively unknown at this time, these terms likely referred to corundum, or white sapphire, as well as transparent rock crystal or other white gems.

In traditional literature, the diamond has been attributed to curing insanity, epilepsy, and counteracting poisons. This mighty gemstone has been thought of as invincible, able to overcome all temptations and overpower all evil. Diamonds instill all the virtues, grant psychic vision, and are often credited for healing all maladies. The extraordinary brilliance and unsurpassed durability of diamond typically associates it with the sun in many astrological traditions.

In ayurvedic astrology, the diamond is the gemstone of Venus, which accounts for its use in engagement rings. Indeed, the diamond has long been considered to impart fidelity, faith, and constancy in love and in friendship. It is a stone that strengthens bonds, grants courage, and accesses the wisdom of the sages. As a costly and precious stone, many sources ascribe to it qualities relating to wealth, abundance, and power.

Diamond was too hard to be cut by ancient lapidary technology; however, references in ancient Chinese, Arabic, and Hebrew texts refer to the use of diamonds to cut, carve, and etch other gemstones. Over time, when the development of tools reached a level of sophistication that would allow them to cut diamond, faces could be polished, especially given that they followed the natural planes of the stone. To cut in any other direction, the diamond would need to be sawed, a process likely to have taken months for a single stone.[4] India supplied virtually all of the stones in the ancient world up until the seventeenth century, when diamonds were discovered in Brazil.

Today, the major sites where diamonds are mined include India, South Africa, Brazil, Tanzania, Zaire, Angola, Sierra Leone, Venezuela, Borneo, Russia, China, and the United States.[5] Several other African nations are also producers of today's diamonds. Roughly one out of every five diamonds of suitable size is of satisfactory quality for the jewelry trade. Specimens of lowest quality are reserved for industrial purposes, such as abrasives and saws.

Today, diamonds reserve their place as the most precious of all gemstones in the jewelry industry. They are surprisingly more abundant in the earth than generally believed, and the industry preserves their scarcity by locking surplus stones away, thereby maintaining an artificially high price on good-quality gemstones.

Diamonds out-sparkle nearly all other gems. Their allure has kept them in fashion for several centuries. The diamond engagement ring is but one of many standard images called to mind when you are asked to think of this gemstone. Diamonds are, for many, an ideal of perfection, invincibility, radiance, and enlightenment, and their message for the people of our planet is both timely and timeless.

DIAMOND AS AN ARCHETYPE:
THE UNCONQUERABLE

Diamond is most clearly connected to the archetype of invincibility in both ancient and modern literature. Its hardness is entangled with its very identity; no stone has a name that implies such dominion over all other stones as the diamond. This brilliant gemstone outshines other gems as well as being resistant to being cut by them. The notion that diamond was unconquerable, or, more accurately, unpolishable, gave rise to many of its traditional associations, starting with its name, as we have seen. The stone perplexed the ancients specifically because it was indomitable and did not yield to the lapidary's tools. Instead, the diamond was used to conquer other gemstones. Carving tools that make use of the king of gems have been described in thousand-year-old texts as resembling a pen or stylus with a diamond inset at the tip. In the Victorian era, which began shortly after the time when diamonds were first cut and polished, the tradition of diamond's invincibility continued with rings set with natural octahedral diamonds, which were intended for scribbling love notes onto glass.[6]

Using the principles of sympathetic resonance, to possess such an unyielding gemstone was widely thought to grant equal invulnerability to its owner. The solar energy ascribed to diamonds represents success in all endeavors, and the invincible, uncuttable gemstone was believed to bring success, victory, wealth, and happiness to anyone who wore it.

Building a New Foundation

The origin of diamond's unconquerable strength lies in its composition. Diamonds are merely one of several crystalline forms of carbon that occur naturally. In most cases, carbon readily joins with other elements like oxygen and a metallic base to form minerals such as carbonates. In other cases it intermingles with the right mix of ingredients to create organic compounds. Carbon itself is a lightweight element; its atomic number of 6 renders it much lighter, and generally softer, than most other elements. When all the conditions are just right, however, carbon atoms align themselves in distinctly cubic arrangements, with all the members of the crystal lattice compacted together, sharing covalent bonds. The end result is a very dense, crystalline form of carbon: the diamond. Diamonds form under intense conditions and are often found in the igneous rock kimberlite, in the hearts of once-active volcanoes, or in the cores of ancient stars. Diamonds may be extremely hard but they are not impermeable; they can be split along certain planes of cleavage, rather like the grain of wood. Certain forms of diamond are also much tougher than others, with octahedral crystals being the hardest.

The cubic crystal family shares many traits, and two of its members have already been encountered on our journey: lazurite and pyrite, both found in lapis lazuli. Like these two minerals, diamond has a crystal lattice that yields cubes as well as a number of related forms governed by the same internal geometry. The most common form is the octahedron, one of the Platonic solids; it resembles two four-sided pyramids attached base-to-base. Diamonds may also be six-sided, twelve-sided, and upward, with some crystals exhibiting 52 faces. All cubic minerals have three axes of symmetry that are of equal length and meet at right angles to one another. No other crystal system exemplifies as much symmetry and congruency as cubic crystals. Another term for this system is *isometric,* meaning "equal measure" because of the regularity of the dimensions. Cubic minerals convey this sense of order, regularity, and simplicity in their energies, and the diamond is perhaps one of the best examples.

Isometric stones resemble building blocks when magnified; tiny cubes or other regular shapes are stacked together to make minerals that are often very dense. They are logical, direct, and often grounded. They act like bricks in that they build up a framework for whatever goal to which they are applied. When a diamond is worn for health, for example, it goes to the most basic level of manifestation on which the desired result exists, and from there it begins to restructure the framework of one's wellness. Diamonds work similarly on the mental, emotional, and spiritual levels, too.

When diamond is used in any given scenario it brings indelible, inarguable, unchanging order to the energy present. Its brilliance and durability penetrate even the most rigid patterns, and it carves away any beliefs or energies that do not support the mission at hand. Simultaneously, diamond's rigidity imposes structure, order, and harmony on the makeup, both physical and subtle, of the situation. When diamond has finished its work, the effects are long-lasting because of the inherent strength achieved with so much order and regularity.

The primary message of the diamond is that of strength. Not a single natural gemstone competes with the strength of diamond, and this invincibility was perceived and admired since antiquity by those lucky enough to meet this stone. Diamond engenders similar qualities in its bearers: unsurpassed strength, incomparable brightness, and an indomitable spirit.

Divine Will

In the esoteric teachings of the seven rays, some systems, such as that of Alice Bailey and Michel Coquet, appoint diamond as the representative gemstone of the first ray of the will. This ray is characterized by "dynamic one-pointedness" and indomitable strength of will.[7] The first ray can be both constructive and destructive, and it carries an extraordinary sense of authority. As the gemstone counterpart to this frequency, the diamond can sometimes seem ruthless and unyielding. It connects to the highest light, and it represents an incarnation of the divine will on the earth plane.

Diamond is a difficult teacher; unlike other gemstones it conveys all the color rays of gemstone therapy and resonates at the most primal level of order. In fact, the diamond is to order what obsidian is to chaos; this shining stone carries the frequency of light and structure into its surroundings. Along the path of the archetypes through which we've journeyed so far, one of the key themes of the journey has been surrender and relinquishment of ego. Whereas stones such as jade and obsidian are gentle nudges toward mastery of this goal, diamond approaches it with exigency and cold detachment. The tone of diamond is one of submission without subjugation; quite simply it breaks down the egoic state without judgment or derision.

Diamond's nature includes both destruction and creation. As the unconquerable stone, it is symbolic of the will of God in that it cannot be swayed or broken by any other force. Similarly, diamond is capable of cutting all other stones, much the way other states of resonance must be shaped by or come into alignment with divine will. The astrological connection to the sun represents the link diamonds have to the solar Logos. In contrast to the crystal sun, as represented by quartz, diamond is the source of the light rather than merely the lens that focuses it on the receiver. Diamond's brilliance and luster are enough to outperform nearly all other gems, optically speaking. This radiance is akin to the light of Source; it outshines all other forces in the universe, because they are all really a part of Source.

Diamond, as the archetype of invincibility, cuts through illusion, ego, and the personality. It replaces human will with divine will in perfect alignment. The orderly nature of diamond's structure and the relative purity of its carbon represent the perfection of the divine will, and it helps to reconstruct our beings in total alignment with Source. When the human ego begins to dissolve, the nature of the soul expresses itself through service, helping it to accomplish its divine purpose on the earth.

Love Conquers All

When diamond is used as a tool for spiritual unfoldment and self-actualization, it slices through all that remains of attachment and will. The power of diamond is sharp, blazing, and ever-victorious. Connecting with diamond reroutes our soul's expression away from personal will and toward divine will, which is singularly expressed through divine love. Every level of manifestation in existence is a manifestation of the expression of the love of Creator. Diamond circumvents ego and personal will, and it connects directly to the unifying principle holding the entire universe together.

Diamonds are also a product of the expression of the divine love. Unlike human beings, diamonds, like other gemstones, never waver from their path or their purpose. Diamond serves as an anchor and entry point for divine love to be made physical. Love exists in many expressions, but it never fails to lose its identity in any form. Sentient beings interpret love differently though its multitudinous channels and countenances; the reality is that the only true love is love without conditions, since conditions and limitations, both products of fear, belong to the ego.

Diamond brings will and love into a perfect coexistence. Together, they are what the famed magician Aleister Crowley mean in his injunction "Do what thou wilt shall be the whole of the Law. Love is the Law, Love under Will." Diamond's vibration is so radically loving that it perfectly aligns love and will into a singular expression of divinity; only the holy will and love exist in harmony with all of creation. Because diamond is so single-pointed in this focus, it tends to strip away any of our limiting beliefs and emotions.

Diamond occurs throughout the universe as one of the very first minerals to occur in the unfolding of history. As exploding stars give up their constituent elements, carbon atoms join together in a crystalline expression of the harmony of the spheres. Given their purity, regularity, and congruent axes, angles, and faces, diamonds give perfection an identity in mineral form. This crystallization is the manifestation of the divine love and will of the universal Logos; through the act of love was our world created, and with it came diamonds.

Because diamonds are in and of themselves supreme manifestations of unconditional love, they can teach us to more purely express the highest form of divine love on all levels of our being. When we do this, there is no force that can throw us off track because no frequency is greater than love. Through this transmission of divine love we become impervious to all external influences. Love is a seed already latent in our beings, and it merely needs light to grow to its potential. Diamond, as the king of gemstones, teaches the human kingdom the true nature of love without conditions or expectations. This, in turn, frees us from attachment, pain, and ego, granting a level of invincibility to our presence in all planes of existence.

Just as carbon, a relatively soft and light element, is changed into the dense and indestructible diamond, love transforms our hearts, tender and fragile as they appear, into inviolable and adamantine vehicles of healing. Diamond may at first seem destructive in that it cuts through the lesser vibrations, but it quickly shines its light so brightly as to illumine the true nature of our being. This flash of brilliance is the moment of crystallization wherein the lightning strike of unconditional love catalyzes our transformation so that we, too, become crystalline.

MEDITATION

ADAMANTINE LIGHT

In a perfect world, each of you reading this book would have access to a flawless diamond to use during these meditations. Because of the prohibitive cost of obtaining such a tool, many of you will be unable to do so. The meditations in the chapter have been written with this in mind, so physical diamonds are not necessary to perform them. Faceted gemstones set in jewelry can be used, although they work best when set alone, without any other accompanying gems. Also, try exploring the list of related stones at the end of this chapter; one of the more accessible stones listed there may appeal to you for use in these meditations.

Begin by holding your diamond in your nondominant hand while standing. As you inhale, visualize the energy of diamond traveling up this arm and into your entire body. As you exhale, allow it to expand beyond your physical body. Repeat this several times until this adamantine light is thoroughly incorporated.

Next, imagine that the energy of diamond is intentionally seeking out your weaknesses or perceived flaws. Each of these is like a crack in the matrix of light surrounding and flowing through you. Diamond seals the cracks with more light, healing and repairing your energy makeup with divine love. With each piece of your being that is restored to perfection you become stronger and invincible.

When you have attained a level of completion, thank the diamond for its work, and briefly contemplate the nature of unconditional love. Know that this is the force now supporting and strengthening you and your energy field; nothing can overturn the power of love.

DIAMOND AS AN ARCHETYPE: THE THUNDERBOLT

In ancient literature, diamond shares names with several other substances and phenomena. In the wisdom teachings of the Vedas as well as in the subsequent Buddhist sutras, the force of enlightenment was traditionally described as *vajra,* which means both "thunderbolt" and "diamond." This concept would be translated into many Asian languages with the spread of Buddhism; the Chinese, Koreans, and Japanese, among others, used *lightning* or *vajra* to imply "diamond" and "indestructible."

In Vedic scripture, the god Indra is frequently depicted holding a vajra; accordingly, several of his epithets incorporate this word. Indra is considered to be the king of the gods as well as having dominion over weather and warfare. The club-shaped implement he holds is the symbol of the thunderbolt wielded by this warrior. It is swift, and few can endure it. Later representations of the vajra found their way into other Asian spiritual traditions.

The vajra features prominently in Mahayana Buddhism, especially in the Vajracchedika Prajnaparamita Sutra, better known as the Diamond Sutra. The Diamond Sutra advocates nonattachment and cultivating without attainment. It seeks to better the student not only for him- or herself but for all sentient beings. The choice of translating *vajra* as "diamond" refers to the indestructible quality of the teachings and of the mind when it achieves the perfected state. Its association with lightning is not diminished, however, for awakening can take place as quickly and unexpectedly as a bolt of lightning. Diamonds themselves work energetically just as quickly and emphatically as the thunderbolt; working with them opens the mind by releasing attachment, thereby permitting a state of liberation. In tantric Buddhism of the Mahayana a vajra (or *dorje* in Tibetan) is a wandlike ritual implement that symbolizes both the properties of a diamond (indestructibility) and a thunderbolt (irresistible force). It is considered a male force and is used ritually in conjunction with the bell, a feminine symbol.

The primary action of the diamond is to promote a state in which the primal unifying force of the universe, unconditional love, can be understood and expressed in perfect harmony. This sense of awakening to unconditional love is a transpersonal experience, for it transcends ego and personality and works at a soul level. Because of this, diamonds are supreme activators of the crown chakra, which blooms into the thousand-petalled lotus of enlightenment. Diamond realigns, releases impediments to, and illumines the crown center with its perfect expression of the light and splendor of divinity made manifest. This access to the heavenly blueprint is the reason why diamonds are so commonly set into the crowns of royalty; being so close to the crown chakra awakens and expands this center of higher consciousness, metaphorically enabling political leaders to make enlightened decisions.

The Diamond Vehicle

One of the three vehicles or paths to enlightenment in Buddhism is known as the Vajrayana, the "diamond vehicle" or "diamond path," also known as tantric Buddhism (the other two paths being the Hinayana and the Mahayana). Although the sense of the adamantine perfection of diamond lends a picture of strength and clarity to the esoteric lore of this path, the message is incomplete without also examining the meaning of the thunderbolt. The actual process of awakening, or attaining enlightenment, may appear to take years, or even lifetimes, of dedicated study and practice, but in the Vajrayana the initiate can receive the final attainment instantaneously, like a thunderbolt.

The vajra is a ritual tool of contemplation. This double-headed scepter is a sign of authority, like the wand or other imperial regalia, but its dominion is over the spiritual rather than the material planes. The diamond vehicle of Buddhism seeks to enlighten its practitioners so that they can be the way-showers and instructors for all sentient beings, thereby leading them out of the ceaseless pattern of *samsara,* the endless cycle of death and rebirth. The practitioner finds salvation by riding the diamond vehicle into a higher and more rarefied level of consciousness.

Diamond shares many esoteric qualities with quartz. The two stones have many optical properties that dazzled ancient people, and they subsequently have overlapping elements of solar imagery and a connection to our crystalline self, the light body. The diamond is the final attainment of body, mind, and spirit in unified evolution. Diamond is the invincible crystallized expression of divine love. It is therefore a profound teacher of our own evolutionary potential.

The diamond is formed under conditions of extreme, concentrated heat and pressure; the image of amorphous coal metamorphosing into precious diamond under the right conditions is conjured. Diamond is an evolutionary stone because it forms when noncrystalline carbon rearranges itself into a more perfected state. Likewise, these gems train the human consciousness to direct the refabrication of the human being into a crystalline, luminous being—in tantric traditions, the "diamond body." Just as carbon needed a previous form before taking on its indestructible incarnation, we need our current state of being in order to move along the path of spiritual evolution.

Diamond is the mentor in achieving the unconquered, luminous body. Working with diamond prepares our physical body by ushering in light; ultimately, it fills every cell in every tissue of every organ. When we are clarified and radiant, the tiniest push in the right direction can be sufficient for self-actualization as well as for the full activation of the diamond body. Diamond itself may not provide this final activation; however, because it functions as ballast for unconditional love and divine will, diamond can facilitate the necessary experience. Even the smallest diamonds are akin to lightning rods that can attract the focus of bursts of celestial light.

Alpha and Omega

Diamonds first took form billions of years ago; as the elements bursting forth from fading stars collided and eventually cooled, carbon atoms combined into the pinnacle of gemstones. These primal diamonds planted seeds of perfection throughout the universe, serving as the initiation of the cycle we are currently experiencing. Diamonds are the result of eons of maturation occurring in the mineral kingdom. As such, they are sometimes considered to be the most highly evolved gems on the planet.[8] Diamonds are the bookmarks of the eternal, for they are both the first and the final gems created.

The diamond represents the transition from one cycle to another. In an instant an entire lifetime can change. This archetype is similarly illustrated by the thunderbolt. Lighting emerges from the heavens and dissipates in an instant, punctuated by thunder. Wherever lightning lands things are permanently changed: trees are felled, sand and stone are turned into vitreous fulgurites, and homes can be destroyed. The presence of the thunderbolt, lightning's punctuation, is felt in diamond because this gemstone forcefully shares its light for revelation and actualization. Only when one is properly prepared can this be met with successful results.

This role of the diamond is a like cosmic alarm clock. In this case, however, diamond's call doesn't wake us up until we have relinquished everything from the sleeping state of unawareness. The importance of the Diamond Sutra is that it instructs the mind to surrender desire, attachment, and identity from the world of form in order to step into the territory of the formless. In this way diamond reminds us of the formless void of obsidian, because through gradual training and ordering of the mind the nature of formlessness can be contemplated and ultimately understood.

Our journey through the crystal archetypes could very well have ended at quartz. Rock crystal's luminous qualities can achieve many of the same ends as diamond. However, diamond represents the threshold into a new cycle; it is both the conclusion of one phase in spiritual evolution and the opening of an entirely new one. The lightning strike that catalyzes the entire process only occurs in a sensitized state, however. That is why diamond cuts through illusion and ego without mercy.

The diamond is the cutter of all attachments. It shares this blade-like imagery with obsidian. The high value of diamonds in our material plane is part of the illusion that we need to dispel. Diamonds are a representation of the power of the mind to overcome desire and ego, no matter the cost. We finally stop dreaming of the illusory realms, and we step into them as whole, awakened beings.

MEDITATION
___

THE THUNDERBOLT

As before, select a diamond or diamond substitute. Lie down comfortably with the stone above your crown center. Breathe evenly and deeply, and let go of any thoughts. Try to allow your mind to be totally blank.

Next, picture the diamond above your crown. In your mind's eye, visualize it glowing and floating above your crown. Whenever a thought arises, imagine that a miniature bolt of lightning jumps from the diamond to your crown chakra, cutting through your thoughts. Repeat this for as long as the visualization is comfortable.

When you are ready to conclude, imagine breathing in through your crown center. With it comes the light of the diamond, helping to make you luminous and transparent. Take several breaths of diamond light and thank the crystal for its assistance in cutting through the illusory nature of the mind. When you have finished, open your eyes.

DIAMOND AS AN ARCHETYPE:
THE BLUEPRINT

The single idea that underpins all the beliefs about diamonds is their innate perfection with regard to their structure and composition. This purity and regularity accounts for many of diamond's properties, including its hardness, radiance, refractive index, and density. The perfection of diamond is therefore responsible for its associations with invincibility and being unconquerable. Since Creator is a whole, perfect force in the universe, the unconditional love expressed by divine will must also exhibit this same level of harmony.

The divine mind serves as the energetic fabric out which all material objects are fashioned. Before any living being or inanimate object can be experienced in the third dimension, it first exists as an idea in the mind of God. This idea is free of limitation, defect, and attachment. Its only expectation is to receive divine love by merely being. The perfected ideal that exists outside of physical incarnation is considered to be the blueprint. Each individual human being has his or her own blueprint. Chairs and desks have blueprints too, as do animals and plants, rocks and minerals, elements, spiritual forces, and other entities. Blueprints are the fundamental information around which matter and energy are organized in the universe that we can see and experience.

Diamonds connect deeply to the blueprint for a variety of reasons. First, because the blueprint is an idealized state, it expresses divine will and divine love without limitations. There are no mistakes in any prototypic rendering in the universal Logos. Diamond, as a perfect incarnation of these principles, expresses its own blueprint in a manner that is comprehensible to other forms of life. As such, it teaches us to connect to the fabric of our own existence. When this contact has been made, any mental, emotional, or spiritual patterns that inhibit the expression of adamantine perfection can be released and transmuted. Diamond works via the principles of sympathetic resonance to instill an unshakable state of purity and regularity on the nonphysical levels. This translates to better health and well-being at the physical level, too.

The nature of an energetic blueprint consists of expressions of spectrums of vibration, chiefly the seven main color rays, as well as other types of information.[9] These energetic infrastructures for physical existence vibrate in harmony with unconditional love. Diamond cuts through and illuminates the boundaries between the blueprint, which is woven from Creator's love and the expression of this love here on the earth. Diamond carries the seven color rays, especially those of therapeutic quality, and so it can heal by restoring equilibrium. In this way, diamond rectifies imbalances, ameliorates deficiencies to any one or more of the rays, and assists the person in "re-aligning with life affirming vibrations."[10]

As Above, So Below

The structure of diamond echoes the message of working at the blueprint level for healing. The most common form of diamond crystal is the octahedron, the eight-sided figure resembling two pyramids placed base to base. This morphology plants the seed of perfection at the geometric level, which is in itself a blueprint-related function. The pure, crystalline order contained at the molecular level of diamond becomes visible through its outer crystal forms, which are encoded to contain and transmit the highest frequencies of light and consciousness.

All of diamond's crystal forms are predicated on the Platonic solids and other figures that can be expressed in sacred geometry. At the seed-crystal level, diamonds display a cubic crystal system, and that means that their inner arrangement of carbon atoms links together in more or less cubic aggregates. Cubic and octahedral crystals are generally the most prevalent forms that diamond takes, and both of these are also Platonic solids. These polyhedral figures are significant because they are more orderly and regular than any other.

Platonic solids include the tetrahedron, cube (or hexahedron), octahedron, dodecahedron, and icosahedron. Each of these is comprised of faces of equal size, edges of equal length, and angles of equal measure. They are the seed forms for all three-dimensional figures, and they can be stretched and morphed into all the other known crystal forms. Diamonds embody the most regular crystal class; cubic minerals exhibit greater degrees of symmetry than any other. As such, diamond's inherent crystallinity steers toward order and harmonizes the resonant fields it comes in contact with.

Most important of all the crystal forms is the octahedron. It connects diamond to the blueprint through its geometric expression. The octahedron is numerologically significant to the understanding of diamond's mission. First, it is comprised of triangles, which are geometrical adaptations of the number three. Three encourages change, motion, and creation. Threes are important for development because they prevent stagnation.

Next, octahedral diamonds have six vertices. In Vedic texts, six-cornered diamonds were considered to be the most powerful. Six is harmonious with the vibration of love. Six is the union of two triangles, forming the Star of David. This can be seen when transparent diamond crystals are held at the correct angle; the rear triangle can be seen in reverse to the front triangle, and they form a six-pointed optical illusion. Six unites opposites in perfect harmony.

The octahedron is named for its eight sides; it is also square in cross-section. These two numbers convey stability and groundedness. Diamond achieves its role as the anchor for divine love and will through these numerological ideals. Four, which is especially stabilizing, also serves to help the positive changes made by three to take hold. Eight has a message of infinity, for the symbol for infinity is a sideways figure eight. This connection reminds us that diamond anchors a frequency of love that is infinite, without limitation or conditions.

Finally, the octahedron and the cube have twelve edges each. Twelve is a higher expression of the order represented by six. It is loving, spiritual, and balancing. Twelve is the number most frequently associated with perfection, completion, and Christ Consciousness. This number often appears in spiritual texts, and it represents spiritual attainment.

In addition to the numbers encoded in the perfected crystal form of diamond, the shape itself is significant. The bipyramidal form is perfectly symmetrical. The upper pyramid is a perfect mirror of the lower; this is a mineralogical and geometrical embodiment of the esoteric axiom "as above, so below." Diamonds serve as a channel through which divine consciousness is made manifest in physical form. Whatever information resides on the blueprint level, the immaterial level of existence, is relayed into our third-dimensional experience on the physical plane. The very morphology of diamonds is inextricably correlated with transducing the encoded love and will of the blueprint into physical form.

The Carbon Connection

One of the reasons why diamond energy incites such profound changes in human consciousness and biological processes is owed to its composition of pure carbon. Working with diamonds allows for a sympathetic resonance between two carbon-based entities, and it is this carbon-to-carbon transmission that is responsible for diamond's ability to reawaken you to the blueprint underlying your very existence.

Diamonds present themselves in several prototypic and archetypal representations of the blueprint. On a cosmic level, as observed by advanced telescopes, "molecular clouds contain a most unusual carbon atom bonded to a hydrogen atom and three other carbon atoms. Further analysis showed that these immense blobs of gas and dust, which eventually give birth to stars, are full of floating micro-diamonds."[11] Other cosmic diamonds exist, too. Examples of micro-diamonds can be found in some meteorites, and the carbonado diamonds found on Earth may actually have been seeded by extraterrestrial diamonds.

Taking this one step further, diamonds may be responsible for translating the blueprint of living organisms in a very real, biological manner. Hydrogenated diamonds such as those found in the clouds of nebulae were present on Earth billions of years ago. These unique crystals interact with water in precise ways; they cause water to "line up," thereby transferring their intrinsic order into the world around them. These orderly arrangements of carbon and water could have been "caught up" with other compounds, which formed early variants of organic compounds, such as DNA and proteins.[12]

Diamonds have been actively engaged in the evolution of physicality since before life on Earth existed. Rather than inertly carrying blueprint information or impersonally pointing the way back to the blueprint, diamonds are mentors, coaches, and builders. They actively work with the information contained within the archetypal ideal for biological life and arrange the world into order around these instructions. In this way, the diamond is a manifestation of order emerging from chaos, or form emerging from the void.

The carbon structure of diamond is vital to its connection to human evolution. Diamonds represent a "primal gate of light" for the union of the small self and the divine.[13] Because it maintains its identity of invincibility, diamond aligns, builds, and anneals on all levels of manifestation. It floods the physical, mental/emotional, causal, and spiritual planes with indomitable, radiant light. This light is a tool for inciting growth, as well as a function of the growth itself.

However, it is through carbon that diamond "brings the pure universal energy down into physical form, ready to be directed by consciousness."[14] Diamond speaks intimately to incarnated life because of carbon. It can be said to unite the mineral and biological kingdoms through its crystallinity and near-organic composition. Diamonds are special, for they exist outside of limitation; diamonds are the beginning and the end, creators and demolishers. They represent a level of spiritual attainment embodying its own arcane level of initiation and evolution.

Blood Diamonds: Corrupted Blueprints

In the gemstone industry, few stones have the effect that diamonds have to activate human greed. In diamond-producing countries, business practices often condone violence, gore, and torture in the name of profit. Miners of these gemstones are often subjected to unsafe working conditions and must work long hours for little pay. Additionally, sales of diamonds in countries engaged in conflict are frequently used to finance continuing warfare. These stones are called "blood diamonds," "conflict diamonds," and "hot diamonds," among other terms, in order to indicate their controversial origins.

Like all minerals, the crystalline matrix of diamond's makeup serves as an excellent means for storing energy and information on a spiritual level. Imagine the energy of those stones that are mined using unethical practices and sold for the profit of organizations at war with one another. The vibrational effect on such gems is profoundly negative, and this energy often circulates in the jewelry industry. Diamonds are among the most expensive and coveted of gemstones, and greed stands adjacent to these stones in many places.

Since diamonds can be tools for accessing our highest level of consciousness, they may actually be used to help heal the rift experienced through the production of conflict stones. While certification processes exist, thereby helping to limit the number of such gems in the market, it may not be possible to know the origin of your favorite gemstone. Because of this, it is possible to work with the stone in order to access a level of blueprint healing that affects its own matrix, as well as that of all of humanity.

Diamonds evoke the state of Christ Consciousness. Just as the Buddhist bodhisattva vow binds its adherent to work for the benefit of all sentient beings, achieving Christ Consciousness helps one to look at the bigger picture for healing. Diamonds are the masters of cutting through illusion. When our mind is equally adamantine and luminous, we are able to see beyond greed and look into the root of suffering. Diamonds, though they may incite greed in many people, are nevertheless powerful tools for releasing avarice and arrogance for the well-being of others. These states of mind only exist when communication between our highest ideal and our incarnate selves becomes cut off or diminished; diamond serves to restore communication in order to express the integral wholeness of the blueprint.

Connecting with diamonds can help to heal the fabric of the collective human consciousness. Use them to release your own attachments first, because this is the simplest way to benefit others. From there, diamond can help you to connect to the collective subconscious of our planet. It can hone your prayers and help their results crystallize into form. Diamonds are excellent tools for sharing your light with the world and for helping the world to receive the redemptive power of divine grace and the light of Christ Consciousness. In this way, working with diamond can stir the most profound sense of compassion.

Diamond is impersonal in nature. It amplifies the intentions and energies in its immediate surroundings. It is perhaps because of this that the diamond trade is replete with greed and pain. Diamonds are incredibly beautiful, durable, and exceptional gemstones. To obtain a diamond, it is necessary to pay an artificially high price. This presents an opportunity to receive abundance with grace, recognizing that financial wealth is merely a tool for expression of the will. When diamond is directed toward cutting down the egoic will, only the divine will remains, which operates solely to multiply the channels of expression for unconditional love. Consciously choosing to meet diamond on this level of awareness can undo the corrupted blueprints of the blood-diamond trade it otherwise amplifies.

Diamond is capable of working more powerfully and with greater subtlety than any other gemstone. With enough conscientious people offering diamond respect and love, it is possible to connect to diamond's own blueprint, as expressed by each diamond in existence, in order to offer healing and awakening to all diamonds and those who work with them. Diamonds can fuel wars, or they can heal nations; the choice is ours.

MEDITATION

HEALING GREED

Like the previous exercises in this chapter, it is not necessary to work with a physical diamond for this meditation. However, having one present greatly amplifies the effect, and it may be set with any other gemstones without any negative impact on the outcome. Among the substitutes detailed at the end of the chapter, kimberlite is particularly harmonious for this application.

If using a diamond or diamond substitute, hold it in whichever hand is most comfortable. Breathe in slowly and rhythmically as you relax. Shift your awareness to the stone. Try to visualize the number of stops it made on its journey to you: mine to miner, to mine foreman, to buyers, to stonecutters, to jewelers, to distributors, to jewelry store. How many hands has it passed through? How many of them were motivated by survival? By greed? By a sincere love for gemstones?

Ask for the guidance of diamond in blessing, and thank all those people who are responsible for the stone you hold. Imagine the intense, fiery light of diamond flooding each person along its journey; this light transmutes their fears, greed, and any other lower vibration. Diamond cuts through the disharmony and rebuilds patterns of unconditional love in their place.

Now imagine this same bright light expanding from your stone and connecting with each and every diamond on Earth. It connects to those set in jewelry. It connects to the stones not yet mined. It connects to the stones with technological and industrial uses. It connects to the stones still being formed, as well as those that have been broken down and destroyed over eons. Each of these diamonds is gleaming with the luminous beauty of its blueprint and the shared blueprint that oversees all diamonds.

When you have allowed this intention to anchor itself, thank the diamond for all that it has to offer. Return your attention to your breath and slowly return to the room.

Absolute Perfection

Diamonds are examples of one of the greatest mysteries in the mineral kingdom. They are elusive gemstones, even though they predate the formation of planet Earth. The diamond, as the highest representation of order among minerals, conveys a concise message of the explicit order and unity among all parts of creation. The structure of the diamond, being the hardest of all minerals, teaches that through the realization of perfection, which is already encoded in our blueprints, we are invincible.

Diamond consciousness is divine consciousness. The work that this gemstone engages in at the soul level doesn't add or subtract anything from our being. Unlike obsidian, which helps us release what isn't serving our highest potential for growth, diamond cuts away our illusions that we are not perfect. When it illuminates the consciousness, revealing in that light the beauty of our blueprint-level information, we see that we are already perfected beings because we are not separate from Source; like the proverbial "diamonds in the rough" we merely need to be polished to reveal that beauty and perfection.

The diamond is a crystallization of unity consciousness, wherein no separation from Source and from others is perceived. Meditating with a diamond reveals the fabric of our spiritual nature; this is like a vast quilt of frequencies from Source, each of them different expressions of unconditional love. Diamond, through its unrelenting clarity and brightness, opens a window through which the crystalline perfection of our highest levels of existence emerges. Furthermore, diamond shows that we are but pieces of the grander picture.

The carbon atoms of diamond share their electrons in a tightly woven series of covalent bonds. We are like those bits of carbon; when we recognize our place in the entire grid, we see that the bonds between all aspects are indivisible, like the lattice from which diamond is made. Recognizing and reading this reinforces the nature of the human spirit, for we are beloved parts of the whole universe. Stepping into this knowing strengthens our own resolve; through diamond's example, we can each become unconquerable.

DIAMOND IN CRYSTAL HEALING

The literature on diamond healing often paints a picture of miracle cures for every malady. Diamonds are expensive, rare, and beautiful, which inspires those who have worked with them for healing to ascribe their influence to many applications. Sources from antiquity maintain that the indomitable spiritual presence of diamond eradicates illness, oppression, and evil. Each of these effects is truly predicated on its ability to awaken and strengthen our connection to our potential for perfection: the blueprint.

Physically, diamonds manifest as crystals of pure carbon with a cubic crystal class. Carbon is the source of most of our structural form in our physical bodies. Complex arrangements of chemical compounds bearing carbon are responsible for life. The inherent purity and simplicity of the chemical makeup of diamond enables it to encourage purification and distillation of our most idealized physical vehicle. Diamonds encourage healthy growth of new cells and tissues; it has even been suggested that the perfection and order of diamond can stimulate activation of the DNA and regeneration of the cells.[15]

The cubic form of diamond's crystal system invites grounding and body awareness. It is strengthening and stabilizing. For this reason, using a diamond in crystal healing is helpful for conditions of over-activity and underactivity, as diamond seeks equilibrium among all forces and processes in the body. The hardness of the mineral also encourages an overall strengthening and toning of the physical body; this can, in turn, yield more physical strength, fitness, and improved stamina.[16] Diamonds are recommended for dizziness and vertigo, for the thymus gland, for the skeletal system, and for the healing of wounds.[17]

When interacting with our blueprint, diamond often resolves a number of imbalances and illnesses. When the information held at the soul level is not being expressed properly it impacts the entire being. Hence, when diamonds bring clarity to the frequencies we are meant to express, grounding and anchoring them into physicality, they can remediate the conditions we are experiencing. The brain and mind are particularly impacted, particularly because of the cubic nature of dia-monds. This gemstone expresses its crystallinity in a highly organized manner, and this translates to our lives by increasing order and logic, and their expression thereof.

When using diamond for mental and physical applications, bear in mind the potency of this gemstone. Placed at the third eye, it induces a state of mental clarity and can also stimulate the imagination.[18] Diamond's strength and hardness fosters more self-confidence as well as a revitalized persona. When diamond helps to align the lower self to the unconditional love of Source, any belief or emotional pattern that is in conflict with love must be set free. We can be rendered fearless and emotionally stabilized merely through this mechanism of diamond's healing.

The king of gemstones helps to heal the egoic concerns of greed, poverty consciousness, entitlement, pride, and envy. Each of these is a pattern resulting from not staying centered in the flow of unconditional love and not recognizing the inherent perfection and connectedness that each sentient being shares with Source. Diamond can be used to shift this perception because it removes the ego from the equation *when consciously directed*. It is important to remember that diamond's efficacy necessitates a high degree of caution and sincerity when using it in such a therapeutic application.

Since diamonds have taken their place as the centerpiece of the ideal engagement ring, they also represent fidelity, trust, and faith. The legends surrounding diamonds attest to their ability to reconcile spats between lovers and ensure faithfulness in marriage. Diamond works to help resolve feelings of self-worth and lovelessness that are often the seat of emotional disharmony. Because diamond awakens us to the truth of our place in the universe, this revelation helps us treat others with dignity, respect, and love.

Spiritually, diamond may offer the most profound level of healing and integration of all minerals. It helps to inspire feelings of gratitude, wisdom, and communion with the divine in all things. Ancient texts describe diamond as a tool for realizing the state of enlightenment, and this is an omnipresent focus for the energy of diamond. It is said to promote "fusion of the personality and the soul," which we now recognize as the result of being in touch with our blueprint.[19]

Diamond is a stone of attainment and mastery. Ancient sources describe it as leading its wearer toward a state of ecstasy, wherein the consciousness is raised to direct communion with and revelation from the divine.[20] Diamond is protective, inasmuch as nothing is greater than divine love; for this reason it has been described as counteracting the effects of the evil eye, witchcraft, and the presence of demons. In truth, ancient writers depicted diamond's effects of resonating to unconquerable light; no outside force is great enough to tear it down.

Diamond is a stone of absolution and absolutism. It immediately restores harmony between our perfected selves and our expressed self here in the third dimension. Because of this action, it helps to nurture a state of grace and purity; all our mistakes are forgiven when we see our divinity.

In a therapeutic setting, diamond is a valuable tool. It has been suggested that its power magnifies the effects of other stones. Diamond can be used when a client or condition is resistant to other stones being used. Diamond cuts through blockages, removing the limitations we perceive in our healing. Connecting to diamonds is a profoundly healing experience, even if just for the benefit of encouraging the perfect expression of our divine potential.

Natural stones and faceted gems are both efficient tools for healing. Each brings its own character, with the brilliance and luster of cut stones being enough to still the mind and encourage higher states of consciousness. Diamonds can be applied easily during any type of healing work, and if physical examples of diamonds are not affordable, then it is possible to call on the energy of diamonds through visualization.

One of the best times to apply diamonds therapeutically is at the end of a crystal healing session. Their cubic crystal structure anchors and stabilizes all the positive changes that have been incurred during the healing session. Diamonds are extremely powerful tools; use them with respect and integrity. It is absolutely necessary to cleanse and clear them fully between sessions, otherwise they can carry information from one client to the next.

Below are a number of varieties of diamonds, some of which are more affordable than others. Natural stones, small laser-drilled beads, and polycrystalline diamonds (also called "carbonado diamonds") can be used with good results. If even these are difficult to locate, several other stones can be used to connect to the mission of diamond, and these are also detailed at the end of this chapter.

Varieties of Diamond

Black Diamond

The black diamond is the most grounding and shielding of all the diamonds. It centers one's focus during meditation and may help in achieving the "no mind" state. Black diamonds complement the brilliance of white diamonds. They can act as an intermediary tool to help the user work with the unforgiving light of diamond energy; essentially, they step down the energy in a way that is gentler and more compatible with the human state when used in tandem with colorless stones. Additionally, consider using black and white diamonds in pairs, with the black diamond at the earth star chakra, below the feet, and the white or clear diamond above the head at the soul star chakra. This combination is balancing and enlivening; it helps to activate the potential of our crystalline bodies for evolution and enlightenment.

On an emotional level, black diamonds represent the ability to break through our walls and enter where the shadows dwell. They are precision tools, not unlike scalpels; for this reason they require patience and respect.[21] In this way they may serve as a more evolved healing tool than obsidian. Be sure you have worked intimately with obsidian, though, and ultimately with all the other archetypal stones before moving to the black diamond.

Blue Diamond

Blue diamonds are typically colored by the presence of the metalloid chemical element boron. They lend a jovial energy, for the blue ray they carry is akin to the energy used to correct imbalances associated with Jupiter in Vedic astrology. Blue diamonds are truly rare, and the presence of boron fine-tunes diamond's energy. Boron compounds are traditionally used in glass and ceramics to enhance their durability; they are also used to insulate against radioactive materials in nuclear reactors. Blue diamond imparts similar shielding and strengthening properties to our spiritual anatomy. They can enhance the outer layer of the aura to be more resistant to foreign energies and less likely to be punctured to permit the attachment of cords and entities. Blue diamonds are occasionally recommended for health of the male reproductive system, especially any concerns related to the seminal vesicles.[22]

Brown Diamond

Brown diamond is, by far, the most plentiful of all the different colors of diamonds. It is slightly more grounding than other varieties, and it can fortify and strengthen our resolve. Use it for connecting with the different diamond archetypes, although it is not as well-suited to healing at the blueprint level as the other types. Brown diamond does not equally disperse and refract all seven color rays, and it may disrupt the energy anatomy unless used consciously and conscientiously. It can, however, serve as a reminder to enjoy life on earth. Brown diamond supports physicality and can bring joy to the earthly plane.

Carbonado Diamond

Carbonado, sometimes called "black diamond," is an impure, polycrystalline form of natural diamond. It consists of raw diamond, graphite, and amorphous carbon, the mixture of which results in the toughest form of natural diamond. More porous than other varieties, carbonado is typically black or dark gray in color. While there is no clear consensus on its formation, carbonado diamond is considered to be very old, and it may have its origins in meteorites. One study indicates that its source may actually be a supernova that predates the formation of our solar system.

Carbonado diamond is the prototypical diamond. It is the precursor to the diamonds that we know and love, and it is possible that it was formed and brought to Earth even before any terrestrial diamonds existed. This possibility may support the idea that carbonado seeded the consciousness of diamond on our planet, thus paving the way for the evolution of all the kingdoms on planet Earth, beginning with the mineral kingdom. Carbonado diamond is the primal healer, the blueprint of the blueprint. As such, it is extremely powerful because it serves as a direct bridge to the primordial void while maintaining the penetrating crystallinity of the diamond. Carbonado diamond encompasses the entire journey of this text, from the void of obsidian to the order embodied by diamond. Use it with respect and caution.

Green Diamond

Green diamond opens us up to experiencing accelerated growth on the physical level. It occurs only very rarely in nature, and this prized gemstone breaks down the barriers to change when applied in meditation or healing. It cuts through resistance and helps in accessing the level at which fundamental growth occurs. In the physical body it may accelerate cellular growth to facilitate healing and recovery. On the mental-emotional level, green diamond seeks out our vestigial fears and anxieties concerning change so we can surrender to the process of unfolding.

Luminescent Diamond

Of all the permutations of diamond, this stone, which emits light of its own, is the most mystical. A small percentage of diamonds will fluoresce when exposed to UV light, and an even smaller fraction will phosphoresce from exposure to light of varying sources. These were known to the ancient Chinese as *yeh ming zhu, ming yue chu,* and *yeh kuang bi,* meaning "evening bring pearl," "bright moon pearl," and "night shining gem" respectively.[23] It is likely that several other glowing gems in Hellenistic myth may actually have referred to diamonds that became luminous at night.

Diamonds exhibiting fluorescence have a luminescence activated by ultraviolet light. Estimates regarding the total amount of fluorescent diamonds varies widely, from as little as 10 percent of all diamond specimens to as much as 50 percent of stones.[24] The most frequently seen colors of fluorescence include blue, orange, yellow to green, and white, though others are also found infrequently.[25] These may be due to a wide variety of factors, with the commonest being trace amounts of nitrogen and aluminum, including changes resulting from radiation. Fluorescent stones resonate to the revelation of hidden truths. Because they convert invisible ultraviolet light to the narrow band of energy known to us as visible light, fluorescent diamonds can help to translate hard-to-understand spiritual information into simpler terms, while preserving the core concepts. They also impart light, joy, and wonder to those who meditate on them.

Phosphorescent gems literally speak a language of light unlike any other members of the mineral kingdom. If you find a diamond that glows—or any other crystal for that matter—treasure it! It links the earthly self directly to Creator, for it helps us embrace our inner power and our innate light. A glowing diamond may represent the Great Central Sun, and it reminds the soul of its connection to Source, which can never be diminished.

Red and Pink Diamond

These are among the most valuable of colored diamonds, with the most richly saturated hues being rarest. Paler reds and pinks radiate with a softer, more loving energy than most other members of the diamond clan. The intensity of some of the deep red and pink stones is fiery; these stones are not for the faint of heart! They impart an energetic transfer of kundalini energy which may jump-start the evolutionary process. One author writes that this diamond "catapults us to God," conveying the intensity and momentum that these stones carry.[26]

Pink diamonds carry innocence, and they nurture a state of open-heartedness.[27] Connecting with these stones imparts a clear sense of the unconditional love that permeates the fabric of the blueprint from which we are made. They help us gain better perspective, and this provides a glimpse into both inner and outer beauty in all beings and all situations.

Silver Diamond

Raw diamond is often silvery or metallic until polished. Lower-quality stones will be markedly gray in appearance. This gemstone connects us to warrior energy. It unites the archetype of obsidian to the highest spiritual ideal. Gray and metallic stones are overall much gentler than their optically clear cousins, thereby making them excellent as a first diamond in any therapist's toolbox.

Traditional Vedic texts describe silvery, metallic diamond as belonging to the laborer class; because of this connection, silver diamond can be harnessed for increasing physical strength and vitality.[28] It helps in overcoming temptation and distraction, as well as softening the intensity generally associated with diamonds in therapeutic applications.

Yellow Diamond

Yellow diamond, sometimes referred to as "canary," derives its color from trace amounts of nitrogen. Yellow is a plentiful color among untreated diamonds, although saturated, richly colored stones are quite valuable. Considered to "shine like the sun," the yellow variant of the king of gems is profoundly uplifting.[29] It combines the penetrating brilliance of diamond with the cheery, joyful outlook of pure sunshine.

Yellow diamond has a decidedly solar energy, and this connects it to the astrological associations of the sun. Ayurvedic tradition dictates that the yellow diamond was reserved for the merchant class.[30] Wearing yellow diamond can assist in achieving material wealth and prosperity, although it flows from a level of conscious attunement to the true nature of abundance. It can also provide determination, natural beauty, and an increased sense of style.[31]

Related Stones

In light of the exorbitant cost that comes with owning a fine diamond, several alternative stones will be described among the related stones in this section. They may provide a suitable link to the archetypal energies of diamond through focused intention and appropriate programming prior to using in any of the exercises in this chapter.

Cubic Zirconia

Properly, this gem is cubic zirconium oxide, a compound not generally stable enough to be found in nature. Because of this, lab-synthesized stones are stabilized by the addition of yttrium oxide.[32] Optically flawless, durable, and brilliant, this stone makes a suitable substitute for diamond in the jewelry industry. In rare cases it may be found in nature, though not generally in gem-quality deposits. It shares a crystal system with the diamond, although cubic zirconia (CZ) generally has a lower refractive index.

Use of zirconia as a substitute for diamond is available in more than just the gemstone trade. Faceted examples of this gemstone can be used in place of diamond in spiritual endeavors, too. Because it is man-made, it has not had the opportunity to be incubated and taught by Mother Earth during its formation; perhaps by keeping it close to kimberlite and using the two in tandem you can mitigate the "new" feeling of CZ. Treat it respectfully and program it to work specifically on the task at hand. CZ is said to produce a "mercurial joy" as well as lead one to "believe in a world of abundance."[33] Be mindful, however, that CZ can sometimes have a distracting energy.

Fluorite Octahedron

Fluorite is a halide of calcium and fluoride. It forms as many of the same crystal forms of diamond, including cubes and octahedral crystals. Because of the related geometry, fluorite may occasionally serve as a substitute for diamond in meditation. Its hardness is much lower than that of diamond, however, and it is therefore a more diffuse energy overall.

Overall, fluorite has an overly mental energy. It grounds the consciousness and helps us form good habits. Fluorite is often recommended for enhancing spiritual endeavors because violet and blue are its most common colors. Fluorite also addresses the blueprint and structural level of thought forms. Because it is a cubic mineral and because of its calcium content it is often associated with the elements of skeletal health, alignment, and the framework of ideas and concepts. Ideally, use colorless cubes and octahedrons to connect with diamond energy.

Graphite

Graphite is the fraternal twin of diamond; each is an allotrope of native carbon, differing from one another in crystal form. The geometrical arrangement of graphite's carbon atoms results in much weaker bonds. Because of this, graphite is a much softer stone. Graphite also differs from diamond inasmuch as it is among the best materials for conducting electricity. Because of this, it "can be used during healing activities to enhance the energy transfer from a healer, or other minerals, to the subject of the healing."[34]

Graphite is porous and is also prone to breaking along planes of weak covalent bonds, making it able to reduce friction. Use graphite when the odds seem stacked against you; it may help to reduce the obstacles to success, thus "slicking" the way forward. Graphite's porosity can also encourage learning, especially in technical, mathematical, and communication-based fields. It may be a stone to clear the way before advancing to diamond.

Herkimer Diamond

Herkimer "diamonds" are actually prismatic, double-terminated forms of quartz from Herkimer County, New York. These crystals are slightly harder than most varieties of quartz, and they appear more brilliant and luminous, especially when optically clear. Typically, they contain carbon-based inclusions. Several other locales produce similarly shaped crystals, including Oaxaca, Mexico, and Pakistan.

Herkimer diamond is excellent for accessing the dream state. When found in a pristine, nearly ideal crystal shape it may even superficially resemble a diamond crystal. Its overall brilliance and high vibration makes it an excellent substitute for a real diamond. Its clarity lends it to promoting clear vision, stimulating the intuitive senses, and enhancing spiritual endeavors of all kinds. All of the attributes of quartz, as described in the previous chapter, also apply. It is highly sought after for use in healing on all levels.

Jet

Jet is one of the most revered "stones" of European pagan traditions. Jet is an organic gem material comprised mostly of carbon, as it is in reality a lignite coal, the precursor to other, denser types of coal. Jet has been used in ornamentation for millennia, and it was often used in tandem with amber, another organic gem.

Although it is much softer than diamond, jet, too, forms under pressure. It can help remind one that the forces at work in our lives are the process by which we are transformed from coal into crystalline carbon. Jet makes for a grounding stone; it is deeply connected to the earth because it bridges the plant and mineral kingdoms. Use it to support, protect, and comfort new projects.

Kimberlite

Kimberlite is the mother rock of the diamond industry. It is named after the town of Kimberley, in South Africa, where the 1869 discovery of an 83.5-carat (16.70 g) white diamond, the famous Star of South Africa, spawned a diamond rush, eventually creating the Big Hole, said to be the largest hand-excavated open-pit mine in the world.

This igneous rock is the source of many unusual mineral occurrences, although diamonds remain the most treasured of all. Kimberlite is formed more deeply in the earth's mantle than any other known igneous rock, and it is forcibly extruded in pipes, sills, and dykes in which they are mined today. Kimberlites tend to be low in silica, high in metals such as nickel, magnesium, and potassium, as well as higher than most rocks in carbon dioxide. They are an important source for many other minerals.

Kimberlite it a tough, dark rock. It can help to move energies that have been stagnant for great lengths of time. Use it in moderation, however, because it tends to cause rapid, forcible changes not unlike the geological changes resulting in its rise to the surface of the earth. When focused toward emotional well-being, kimberlite is an excellent tool for anyone who bottles emotions or hides their feelings. Keep in mind that a proclivity toward sudden eruption comes with the use of kimberlite.

Shungite

Shungite is a relatively recent addition to the world of healing crystals, although it has been known it its home country for centuries. Shungite is found only near Shunga village, in Karelia, Russia. It is a carbon-bearing rock with a unique composition: it is the only natural, terrestrial source for fullerenes. Named after Buckminster Fuller, fullerenes—which have been dubbed "buckyballs"—are complex carbon molecules forming spheres and tubes and many other shapes. These hollow compounds act as antioxidants, which can slow the growth of cancer cells and the development of some viruses.[35] In addition to carbon, shungite contains nearly the entire periodic table, and it is available in several grades.

This carbon-based rock is a dynamic healing tool. It is one stone that you may never want to take off, once you get your first piece. There is evidence showing that it works on many levels, such as purifying and enlivening water, neutralizing harmful energy fields (especially EMFs), relieving skin conditions, and supporting the electrical processes of the body. It is especially alchemical and alive. Shungite is grounding without ever feeling heavy.

The molecular composition of shungite also makes it ideal for blueprint-level healing such as that experienced with diamond. In fact, it makes a gentle ally when working with diamond in the healing arts because it can be a buffer to the otherwise intense and often harsh energy of the king of gems. Shungite is an evolutionary gem that is here to support our development on all fronts.

Zircon

Zircons are among the oldest gems on Earth. Although zircon is tetragonal instead of cubic, it often forms as a slightly elongated octahedron. It complements diamond energy because its frequency is grounding and dynamic. Zircons are known for having the capacity "for transmuting spiritual energies into the physical plane,"[36] as opposed to many stones with intense spiritual energies that seek to transmute from the physical to the immaterial. Nonetheless, because diamond works at the blueprint level, it also effects change first in the spiritual realm before those shifts take place in the physical dimensions. Because of this similarity, zircon can assist diamond by grounding and making these transformations tangible and available.

CONCLUSION

Gemstones and minerals are regarded as some of the most important tools for spiritual development today. In truth, the connections between the mineral kingdom and the human realm are as ancient as life itself, and this relationship informs much of the practice carried on in modern times. Each of the chapters in this book has described how ancient cultures were empowered and healed by gemstones; it is my sincere wish that readers of this book will benefit from knowledge about the archetypal roles of crystals.

THE SEVEN ARCHETYPES IN REVIEW

For easy reference, I am including a brief summary of the messages of the seven crystals below:

Obsidian: Obsidian starts our journey with the spear archetype, which represents a sharpening of the mind. It grants courage and strength to those who embrace it. The mirror refines and polishes obsidian; it takes the sharpness and strength of the spearpoint and internalizes it. With the mirror, our fears are revealed so that we can gradually release them and see the true self. Finally, obsidian opens us to the void, the unformed, creative potential of the universe. When we embrace the void, we become fearless co-creators.

Jade: The jade group of minerals represents an advancement in

Stone Age technology, and it is just as much an upgrade in our spiritual work, too. With the mask, jade peels away the layers of ego and personality that obsidian highlights and focuses in on. It is an emptying out of our programming and expectations. Jade also reminds us early on in our journey that help is all around us; there is an assortment of beings willing to help us travel through nonordinary reality, thus helping us embrace the immortal nature of our nonphysical identity. Jade is also a vessel or gateway for accessing the celestial realms, for through emptiness one becomes light enough to travel upward and onward. Jade of all types represents the doorway leading to the next level.

Lapis lazuli: The striking blue and glittering inclusions of this rock awaken a deeply rooted longing in the human identity. Connecting to lapis helps to expand and awaken our awareness of our divine heritage. Lapis lazuli deeply connects to themes of the eyes and the vision, helping to remind us that what is most important may not be visible to the eyes alone, but can be felt and expressed by the wisdom of the heart. Finally, lapis lazuli teaches that with knowledge of our divine, cosmic lineage, we must accept our roles as creators and kings. Authority over our own lives is our birthright, and lapis helps us to claim this.

Emerald: The most beguiling of green gemstones anchors our presence within the heart center. It teaches the basic tenets of alchemy, and after mastering these concepts emerald grants passage to the stage in which the inner workings of the alchemical arts take place. The Holy Grail helps us look into the heart center as the crucible for transmuting leaden consciousness into gold. The grail myth also reminds us of the need to restore balance between polarities. Emerald awakens the presence of the Goddess in us all and grants passage into the Edenic state, wherein we reclaim our innocence and connectedness to all.

Amethyst: Amethyst has a special role in the mineral kingdom because it teaches mastery over the lower self through temperance.

This stone initiates a purified state, a compulsory step before achieving the higher stages of spiritual growth. Amethyst leads the way into personal and planetary alchemy; those who engage in these sacred arts become the custodians of the earth and the leaders of the new wave of consciousness. Amethyst ultimately helps us honor the sacredness of the entire planet as a holy space, a temple for honoring Source and transmuting our healing opportunities into realities.

Quartz: The primary theme in quartz's archetypes is one of light. As the wand, it refines the strength and pointedness of obsidian's spearpoint. It offers balance and counterpoint to the divine feminine principle of the grail because it elevates the masculine principle too. The mastery that the wand entails readies the consciousness for the clarity of the lens. The crystal lens focuses, enlightens, and magnifies the esoteric order of the explicate universe. Connecting to the optical message of quartz yields new vision, wherein the connectedness to Source and the holy fire that burns brightly illumines our entire presence. This illumination readies us for the final archetype, which seeks to rarefy and enlighten all aspects of our being. The crystalline body is borne from the light within and the light that emanates from Source.

Diamond: The king of gems speaks a language of invincibility through surrender to divine love. Diamond takes the notion of unconditional love out of the realm of aspiration and crystallizes it into our everyday lives. It leads human consciousness to the brink of enlightenment because it is the hardest, sharpest, most luminous tool the mineral kingdom has to offer. It cuts through any vestiges of fear or illusion, not merely because of the deftness of its incisive qualities, but also because in the presence of perfection imperfection falls away. At this level of organization we can clearly see into the fabric out of which the entire universe is formed. Here is where we initiate all changes and accept our inherently connected, divine nature.

THE BIG PICTURE

The journey from obsidian to diamond parallels the first step we take, in total darkness, toward the goal of complete illumination. At first glance, the first six archetypal gems represent a complete cycle on their own. They begin and end with silica, the first gem being amorphous and the last perfectly crystallized. The spear evolves into the wand, and the optics of mirrors and lenses align effortlessly to come full circle. Although the progression could stop here, the diamond takes us deeper, for it guides us into a new realm.

Obsidian is the stone of initiation. In many mystery traditions the spiritual aspirant must be blindfolded or placed in complete darkness, symbolizing the void and the womb simultaneously. Obsidian, even with its mirror, only reveals the shadow side; it does not shed light on its own, so it can only guide one to the places in need of light. The initiate must feel his or her way through the trials, which requires a state of total surrender. This process involves pure trust, thereby bringing the consciousness into a state of allowing.

The void is the unmanifest potential of unconditional love. This void is chaos incarnate; it is entropy in motion. Obsidian, for its lack of crystal lattice, totally embodies this symbol. The void is pure potential, and all that emerges is an expression of love. On the opposite end of the spectrum, diamond is perfection made manifest. Where obsidian speaks in possibilities, diamond speaks in absolutes.

The perfection and absolutism of diamond sharply contrasts the beginning of the journey through spiritual initiation. Perfection is born through absolution, wherein our weaknesses and flaws are forgiven—a chief mechanism of surrendering to divine love. We recognize our inseparability from Source, and we are accordingly purified. Nothing that is part of the absolute and holy Creator could ever truly be imperfect.

Accordingly, diamond, for all its connotations of promises and fidelity, represents sincere faith. The trust and surrender developed by following obsidian's lead can be transformed into genuine faith in the will and love of the Logos. Seeing oneself as an integral part of the whole yields a crystallization of unity consciousness. This, in turn, endows the practitioner with untold strength, because no external influence is greater than the unconquerable love felt by connecting to Source.

Each member of the mineral kingdom is a spiritual gift to all sentient beings. Although we have only explored a few of the innumerable gemstones and crystals, each resonates as a crystallization of the will of God. Crystals lack personalities, egos, and expectations; they have mastered the art of being. In light of this, quartz never forgets why it came to Earth; it never tries to be calcite or ruby. The mineral kingdom is an effective teacher and model for our spiritual evolution.

In connecting to the crystals in this book, I hope that your practice and perception are both enhanced. Looking past the surface-level interpretation of what crystals offer us is a skill that opens new doors. Experiment with other stones in your toolbox; each one has stories to tell beyond what can be read in books. The crystalline world is open to us, and it is willing to lead the human consciousness to places we cannot even imagine.

NOTES

CHAPTER 1. OBSIDIAN

1. Lecouteux, *Lapidary of Sacred Stones,* 239.
2. Conway, *Crystal Enchantments,* 248.
3. Serrano, *Obsidiana,* 24.
4. Conway, *Crystal Enchantments,* 248.
5. Ibid., 250.
6. Yamaguchi, *Light on the Origins of Reiki,* 86.
7. Raphaell, *Crystal Enlightenment,* 93.
8. Ibid., 94.
9. Brown, *Daring Greatly,* 34.
10. Serrano, *Obsidiana,* 161. Author's translation.
11. Williamson, *Return to Love,* 190.
12. Raphaell, *Crystalline Illumination,* 79.
13. Melody, *Love Is in the Earth,* 515.
14. Simmons and Warner, *Moldavite,* 93.

CHAPTER 2. JADE

1. Keverne, *Jade,* 23.
2. Ibid., 2.
3. Ibid., 26.
4. Chou, *Dictionary of Jade,* 31 and 82.
5. Levy and Scott-Clark, *Stone of Heaven,* 8.
6. Keverne, *Jade,* 216.
7. Chou, *Dictionary of Jade,* 65.
8. Keverne, *Jade,* 217.

9. Johari, *Healing Power of Gemstones,* 177.

10. Bravo, *Crystal Healing Secrets,* 154.

11. Gimbutas, *Language of the Goddess.*

12. Zara, *Jade,* 23.

13. "Chinese Dragon," https://en.wikipedia.org/wiki/Chinese_dragon (accessed June 25, 2016).

14. Zara, *Jade,* 46.

15. Ibid., 67.

16. Ibid.

17. Grant, *Book of Crystal Spells,* 199.

18. Teresa Kennedy, *Gems of Wisdom,* 17; Mégemont, *Metaphysical Book of Gems,* 213.

19. Asar, *Liquid Crystal Oracle,* 162.

20. Kaehr, *Edgar Cayce,* 112.

21. Helferich, *Stone of Kings,* 138.

22. Chase and Pawlik, *Healing with Gemstones,* 125.

23. Dolfyn, *Crystal Wisdom,* 129.

24. Chou, *Dictionary of Jade,* 29.

25. Confucius, in Chocron, *Healing with Crystals,* 70–71.

26. Kennedy and St. Claire, *Crystal Light and Love,* 65.

27. Helferich, *Stone of Kings,* 106.

28. Ibid., 107.

29. Isabelle Morton, "Introducing Green Jade/ Prehnite" (notes from Gemstone Therapy Institute, July 2013).

30. Gienger and Maier, *Healing Stones,* 112.

31. Isabelle Morton, "Introducing Green Jade/ Prehnite" (notes from Gemstone Therapy Institute, July 2013).

32. Hugs, *Handy Little Crystal List,* 98.

33. Heath, *Book of Stones,* 337.

34. David and Van Hulle, *Michael's Gemstone Dictionary,* 78.

35. Dow, *Crystal Journey,* 202.

36. Simmons and Ahsian, *Book of Stones,* 214.

37. Hugs, *Handy Little Crystal List,* 98.

38. Levy and Scott-Clark, *Stone of Heaven,* 113.

39. Group, *Eight Crystal Alliances,* 239; Heath, *Book of Stones,* 336.

40. Hall, *Crystal Bible,* 153.

41. Gienger, *Crystal Power,* 298.

42. David and Van Hulle, *Michael's Gemstone Dictionary,* 202.

43. Simmons and Ahsian, *Book of Stones,* 214.

44. Ibid., 211.

45. David and Van Hulle, *Michael's Gemstone Dictionary,* 83.

46. Zara, *Jade,* 64.

47. Ibid., 67.

48. Hall, *Crystals and Sacred Sites,* 166.

49. Simmons and Ahsian, *Book of Stones,* 213.

50. Dow, *Crystal Journey,* 202.

51. Hall, *Crystal Bible,* 153.

52. David and Van Hulle, *Michael's Gemstone Dictionary,* 203.

53. Hall, *Crystal Bible,* 153; David and Van Hulle, *Michael's Gemstone Dictionary,* 201.

54. Melody, *Love Is in the Earth,* 80.

55. Hall, *Crystal Bible,* 36.

56. Ibid., 37.

57. Sperling, *Essence of Gemstones,* 87.

58. Isabelle Morton, "Introducing Green Jade/ Prehnite" (notes from Gemstone Therapy Institute, July 2013).

59. Simmons and Ahsian, *Book of Stones,* 356.

60. Ibid.

61. Melody, *Love Is in the Earth,* 811.

CHAPTER 3. LAPIS LAZULI

1. Searight, *Lapis Lazuli,* 3.

2. Bakhtiar, *Afghanistan's Blue Treasure,* 115.

3. Ibid., 113.

4. Searight, *Lapis Lazuli,* 5.

5. Bakhtiar, *Afghanistan's Blue Treasure,* 106.

6. Kaehr, *Edgar Cayce,* 164.

7. Bakhtiar, *Afghanistan's Blue Treasure,* 99.

8. Searight, *Lapis Lazuli,* 68.

9. Lecouteux, *Lapidary of Sacred Stones,* 284.

10. Searight, *Lapis Lazuli,* 54.

11. Kunz, *Curious Lore,* 37.

12. Bakhtiar, *Afghanistan's Blue Treasure,* 70.

13. Michael Katz, *Gemstone Energy,* 206.

14. Bakhtiar, *Afghanistan's Blue Treasure,* 23.

15. Searight, *Lapis Lazuli,* 21.

16. Kunz, *Curious Lore,* 229.

17. Searight, *Lapis Lazuli,* 47.

18. Ibid.

19. Michael Katz, *Gemstone Energy,* 206.

20. Searight, *Lapis Lazuli,* 155.

21. Kunz, *Curious Lore,* 104.

22. Searight, *Lapis Lazuli,* 37.

23. Ibid., 117.

24. Kozminsky, *Magic and Science,* vol. 2, 18.

25. Calverly, *Crystal Yoga,* 71.

26. Bakhtiar, *Afghanistan's Blue Treasure,* 33.

27. Searight, *Lapis Lazuli,* 109.

28. Trask, *12 Gemstones,* 35.

29. Ibid.

30. Pelikan, *Secrets of Metals,* 220.

31. Walker, *Book of Sacred Stones,* 144.

32. Johari, *Healing Power of Gemstones,* 178.

33. Gurudas, *Gem Elixirs,* 122.

34. Michael Katz, *Gemstone Energy,* 208.

35. Roeder, *Crystal Co-Creators,* 118.

36. Simmons and Ahsian, *Book of Stones,* 228.

37. Ibid., 64.

38. Ibid., 63.

39. Sperling, *Essence of Gemstones,* 157.

40. Ibid., 158.

CHAPTER 4. EMERALD

1. Lecouteux, *Lapidary of Sacred Stones,* 297.

2. Ibid., 298.

3. Adapted by the author from several translations.

4. Hauck, *Emerald Tablet*, 52.

5. Ibid., 54.

6. Gienger, *Crystal Power*, 114.

7. Melchizedek, *Ancient Secret*, 170.

8. Murphy, *Gemstone*, 33.

9. Ibid., 35.

10. Caldecott, *Crystal Legends*, 140.

11. Murphy, *Gemstone*, 174.

12. Simmons and Warner, *Moldavite*, 100.

13. Murphy, *Gemstone*, 38.

14. Morgan, *From Satan's Crown*, 10.

15. Ibid., 53.

16. Ibid., 54.

17. Coquet, *Stones of the Seven Rays*, 121.

18. Ibid., 157.

19. Caldecott, *Crystal Legends*, 145.

20. Murphy, *Gemstone*, 13.

21. Morgan, *From Satan's Crown*, 82.

22. Ibid.

23. Walker, *Book of Sacred Stones*, 123.

24. Navran, *Jewelry*, 112.

25. Simmons, *Stones*, 220.

26. Michael Katz, *Gemstone Energy*, 56.

27. Ibid., 59.

28. Gienger, *Crystal Power*, 125.

29. Michael Katz, *Aquamarine Water*, 6.

30. Melody, *Love Is in the Earth*, 102.

31. Sperling, *Essence of Gemstones*, 105.

CHAPTER 5. AMETHYST

1. Dibble, *Quartz*, 37.

2. Dake, Fleener, and Wilson, *Quartz Family*, 86.

3. Trask, *12 Gemstones*, 151.

4. Kozminsky, *Magic and Science*, vol. 1, 97.

5. Isaacs, *Gemstones*, 77.

6. Fairchild, *Crystal Masters,* 192.

7. Michael Katz, *Gemstone Energy,* 248.

8. Fairchild, *Crystal Masters,* 184.

9. Prophet and Prophet, *Masters,* 544.

10. Ibid., 313.

11. Dake, Fleener, and Wilson, *Quartz Family,* 87.

12. Raphaell, *Crystalline Transmission,* 174.

13. Ibid., 179.

14. Dow, *Crystal Journey,* 137.

15. Randazzo, *Rock-Medicine,* 41.

16. Raphaell, *Crystal Enlightenment,* 79.

17. Michael Katz, *Gemstone Energy,* 249.

18. Leavy, *Auralite-23,* 41.

19. Ibid, 177.

20. Twintreess, *Stones Alive! 2,* 187.

21. Melody, *Love Is in the Earth,* 751.

22. Ibid., 752.

23. Ibid.

24. Twintreess, *Stones Alive! 2,* 191.

25. Katz and Katz, *Gifts,* 117.

26. Ibid., 119.

27. Sperling, *Essence of Gemstones,* 357.

CHAPTER 6. QUARTZ

1. Dibble, *Quartz,* 7.

2. Dorland, *Holy Ice,* 155.

3. DeSalvo, *Power Crystals,* 39.

4. Raulet and Boucheron, *Rock Crystal,* 84.

5. Baer and Baer, *Windows of Light,* 17.

6. Raphaell, *Crystal Healing,* 176.

7. Ibid., 175.

8. Temple, *Crystal Sun,* 35.

9. Baer and Baer, *Crystal Connection,* 96.

10. Temple, *Crystal Sun,* 108.

11. DeSalvo, *Power Crystals,* 36.

12. Dorland, *Holy Ice,* 75.

13. Temple, *Crystal Sun,* 273.

14. Ibid., 97.

15. Raulet and Boucheron, *Rock Crystal,* 46.

16. Ibid.

17. Ibid., 25.

18. Temple, *Crystal Sun,* 103.

19. Ibid.

20. Ibid., 106.

21. Ibid., 299.

22. Tag, *Das geheimnis,* 286–89.

23. Temple, *Crystal Sun,* 220.

24. Dorland, *Holy Ice,* 4.

25. Kunz, *Curious Lore,* 227.

26. Tag, *Das geheimnis,* 160.

27. Raulet and Boucheron, *Rock Crystal,* 159.

28. Baer and Baer, *Crystal Connection,* 18.

29. Simmons, *Stones,* 8.

30. Ibid.

31. Ibid.

32. Ibid., 33.

33. Michael Katz, *Gemstone Energy,* 51.

34. Melody, *Love Is in the Earth,* 555.

35. Simmons and Ahsian, *Book of Stones,* 276.

36. Raphaell, *Crystal Healing,* 143–53.

37. Dow, *Crystal Journey,* 255.

38. Michael Katz, *Gemstone Energy,* 333.

CHAPTER 7. DIAMOND

1. Harlow, *Nature, of Diamonds* 13

2. Maillard, *Diamonds,* 194.

3. Wright and Chadbourne, *Gems,* 2.

4. Maillard, *Diamonds,* 199.

5. Ibid., 186.

6. Conway, *Crystal Enchantments,* 81.

7. Coquet, *Stones of the Seven Rays,* 195.

8. Lorusso and Glick, *Healing Stoned,* 35.

9. Ginny Katz, *Beyond the Light,* 59; Isabelle Morton, "Introducing Diamond Therapy" (teleseminar, Gemstone Therapy Institute, April 10, 2015).

10. Kaehr, *Edgar Cayce,* 122.

11. Dorland, *Holy Ice,* 82.

12. Simmons, *Stones,* 81.

13. Ibid., 179.

14. Silver, *Jewels,* 154.

15. Kaehr, *Edgar Cayce,* 122.

16. Twintreess, *Stones Alive!,* 69.

17. Ibid.; Group, *Eight Crystal Alliances,* 201.

18. Hall, *101 Power Crystals,* 80.

19. Group, *Eight Crystal Alliances,* 201.

20. Cunningham, *Cunningham's Encyclopedia,* 92.

21. Sperling, *Essence of Gemstones,* 117.

22. Costelloe, *Complete Guide,* 148

23. Laufer, *Diamond,* 56–57.

24. Warren and Gleason, *Ultraviolet Light,* 194.

25. Ibid.

26. Sperling, *Essence of Gemstones,* 116.

27. Costelloe, *Complete Guide,* 191.

28. Coquet, *Stones of the Seven Rays,* 191.

29. Sperling, *Essence of Gemstones,* 113.

30. Coquet, *Stones of the Seven Rays,* 191.

31. Costelloe, *Complete Guide,* 209.

32. Lyman, *Simon and Schuster's Guide,* 338.

33. Sperling, *Essence of Gemstones,* 377.

34. Melody, *Love Is in the Earth,* 302.

35. Martino, *Shungite,* 33–37.

36. Simmons and Ahsian, *Book of Stones,* 435.

BIBLIOGRAPHY

Asar, Justin Moikeha. *Liquid Crystal Oracle*. Victoria, B.C.: Blue Angel Publishing, 2010.

Baer, Randall N., and Vicki V. Baer. *The Crystal Connection: A Guidebook for Personal and Planetary Ascension*. New York: Harper and Row, 1987.

———. *Windows of Light: Quartz Crystals and Self-Transformation*. New York: Harper and Row, 1984.

Bakhtiar, Lailee McNair. *Afghanistan's Blue Treasure: Lapis Lazuli*. [n.p.]: Front Porch Publishing, 2012.

Bravo, Brett. *Crystal Healing Secrets*. New York: Warner Books, 1988.

Brown, Brené. *Daring Greatly: How the Courage to Be Vulnerable Transforms the Way We Live, Love, Parent, and Lead*. Garden City, N.Y.: Avery, 2015.

Caldecott, Moyra. *Crystal Legends: Stories of Crystals and Gemstones in Myth and Legend*. Bath, U.K.: Mushroom eBooks, 2000.

Calverley, Roger. *Crystal Yoga 1: The Crystal Mesa*. Twin Lakes, Wis.: Lotus Press, 2006.

Chase, Pamela Louise, and Jonathan Pawlik. *Healing with Gemstones*. Franklin Lakes, N.J.: Career Press, 2002.

Chocron, Daya Sarai. *Healing with Crystals and Gemstones: Balance Your Chakras and Your Life*. San Francisco: Red Wheel/Weiser, 2005.

Chou, Mark. *Dictionary of Jade Nomenclature*. Hong Kong: New Island Printing Co., 1987.

Conway, D. J. *Crystal Enchantments: A Complete Guide to Stones and Their Magical Properties*. Berkeley, Calif.: Crossing Press, 2000.

Coquet, Michel. *Stones of the Seven Rays: The Science of the Seven Facets of the Soul*. Rochester, Vt.: Destiny Books, 2012.

Costelloe, Marina. *The Complete Guide to Crystal Astrology: 360 Crystals and*

Sabian Symbols for Personal Health, Astrology and Numerology. Findhorn, Moray, Scotland: Findhorn Press, 2007.

Cunningham, Scott. *Cunningham's Encyclopedia of Crystal, Gem and Metal Magic.* St. Paul, Minn.: Llewellyn Publications, 1994.

Dake, H. C., Frank L. Fleener, and Ben Hur Wilson. *Quartz Family Minerals: A Handbook for the Mineral Collector.* New York: Whittlesey House, 1938.

David, Judithann, and J. P. Van Hulle. *Michael's Gemstone Dictionary.* Orinda, Calif.: Affinity Press, 1990.

DeSalvo, John. *Power Crystals: Spiritual and Magical Practices, Crystal Skulls, and Alien Technology.* Rochester, Vt.: Destiny Books, 2012.

Dibble, Harold L. *Quartz: An Introduction to Crystalline Quartz.* Angola, N.Y.: Dibble Trust Fund, 2003.

Dolfyn. *Crystal Wisdom: Spiritual Properties of Crystals and Gemstones.* Decatur, Ill.: Earthspirit, 1989.

Dorland, Frank. *Holy Ice: Bridge to the Subconscious.* St. Paul, Minn.: Galde Press, 1992.

Dow, JaneAnn. *Crystal Journey: Travel Guide for the New Shaman.* Santa Fe, N.Mex.: Journey Books, 1996.

Fairchild, Alana. *Crystal Masters 333: Initiation with the Divine Power of Heaven and Earth.* Woodbury, Minn.: Llewellyn Publications, 2014.

Gienger, Michael. *Crystal Power, Crystal Healing.* London: Cassell Illustrated, 2009.

———, and Wolfgang Maier. *Healing Stones for the Vital Organs: 83 Crystals with Traditional Chinese Medicine.* Rochester, Vt.: Healing Arts Press, 2009.

Gimbutas, Marija. *The Language of the Goddess.* San Francisco: Harper and Row, 1989.

Grant, Ember. *The Book of Crystal Spells: Magical Uses for Stones, Crystals, Minerals . . . and Even Sand.* Woodbury, Minn.: Llewellyn Publications, 2013.

Group of 5. *The Eight Crystal Alliances: The Influence of Stones on the Personality.* Berkeley, Calif.: North Atlantic Books, 2011.

Gurudas. *Gem Elixirs and Vibrational Healing,* Vol. 1. San Rafael, Calif.: Cassandra Press, 1985.

Hall, Judy. *The Crystal Bible: A Definitive Guide to Crystals.* Alresford, Hampshire, UK: Godsfield Press, 2003.

————. *Crystals and Sacred Sites: Use Crystals to Access the Power of Sacred Landscapes for Personal and Planetary Transformation*. Beverly, Mass.: Fair Winds Press, 2012.

————. *101 Power Crystals: The Ultimate Guide to Magical Crystals, Gems, and Stones for Healing and Transformation*. Beverly, Mass.: Fair Winds Press, 2011.

Harlow, George E., ed. *The Nature of Diamonds*. Cambridge, U.K.: Cambridge University Press, 1998.

Hauck, Dennis William. *The Emerald Tablet: Alchemy for Personal Transformation*. New York: Penguin, 1999.

Heath, Maya. *The Book of Stones and Metals*. Independence, Mo.: Merlyn Press, 2000.

Helferich, Gerard. *Stone of Kings: In Search of the Lost Jade of the Maya*. Guilford, Conn.: Lyons Press, 2011.

Hugs, Kristi (Mira Bai). *The Handy Little Crystal List Reference Guide*. Charleston, S.C.: CreateSpace, 2013.

Isaacs, Thelma. *Gemstones, Crystals, and Healing*. Black Mountain, N.C.: Lorien House, 1987.

Johari, Harish. *The Healing Power of Gemstones: In Tantra, Ayurveda, and Astrology*. Rochester, Vt.: Destiny Books, 1996.

Kaehr, Shelley. *Edgar Cayce Guide to Gemstones: Minerals, Metals, and More*. Virginia Beach, Va.: A.R.E. Press, 2005.

Katz, Ginny. *Beyond the Light: A Personal Guidebook for Healing, Growth, and Enlightenment*. Gresham, Ore.: Golden Age Publishing, 1992.

————, and Michael Katz. *Gifts of the Gemstone Guardians*. Gresham, Ore.: Golden Age Publishing, 1989.

Katz, Michael. *Aquamarine Water: Fountain of Youthful Vitality*. Portland, Ore.: Gemisphere, 2002.

————. *Gemstone Energy Medicine: Healing Body, Mind, and Spirit*. Portland, Ore.: Natural Healing Press, 2005.

Kennedy, Maiya, and Mary St. Claire. *Crystal Light and Love: The Spiritual Reality of Crystal Healing*. Murray, Utah: Inner Mind Publishing, 1988.

Kennedy, Teresa. *Gems of Wisdom, Gems of Power: A Practical Guide to How Gemstones, Minerals, and Crystals Can Enhance Your Life*. Boston: DaCapo Press, 2007.

Keverne, Roger, ed. *Jade: with Over 600 Photographs of Jades from Every Continent*. London: Lorenz Books, 2011.

Kozminsky, Isidore. *The Magic and Science of Jewels and Stones*. 2 vols. San Rafael, Calif.: Cassandra Press, 1988, 1989.

Kunz, George Frederick. *The Curious Lore of Precious Stones*. New York: Dover Publications, 1971.

Laufer, Berthold. *The Diamond: A Study in Chinese and Hellenistic Folk-Lore*. [n.p.] CreateSpace, 2015.

Lecouteaux, Claude. *A Lapidary of Sacred Stones: Their Magical and Medicinal Powers Based on the Earliest Sources*. Rochester, Vt.: Inner Traditions, 2012.

Leavy, Ashley. *Auralite-23: Transformational Amethyst from the Cave of Wonders*. [n.p.] CreateSpace, 2014.

Levy, Adrian, and Cathy Scott-Clark. *The Stone of Heaven: The Secret History of Imperial Green Jade*. London: Weidenfield and Nicolson, 2001.

Lorusso, Julia, and Joel Glick. *Healing Stoned: The Therapeutic Use of Gems and Minerals*. Albuquerque, N.Mex.: Brotherhood of Life, 1984.

Lyman, Kennie, ed. *Simon and Schuster's Guide to Gems and Precious Stones*. New York: Simon and Schuster, 1986.

Maillard, Robert, ed. *Diamonds: Myth, Magic, and Reality*. New York: Crown Publishers, 1988.

Martino, Regina. *Shungite: Protection, Healing, and Detoxification*. Rochester, Vt.: Healing Arts Press, 2014.

Megémont, Florence. *The Metaphysical Book of Gems and Crystals*. Rochester, Vt.: Healing Arts Press, 2008.

Melchizedek, Drunvalo. *The Ancient Secret of the Flower of Life*, Vol. 1. Flagstaff, Ariz.: Light Technology Publishing, 1998.

Melody. *Love Is in the Earth: The Crystal and Mineral Encyclopedia—The LIITE Fantastic and the Last Testament*. Wheat Ridge, Colo.: Earth Love Publishing House, 2008.

Morgan, Diane. *From Satan's Crown to the Holy Grail: Emeralds in Myth, Magic, and History*. Westport, Conn.: Praeger, 2007.

Murphy, G. Ronald. *Gemstone of Paradise: The Holy Grail in Wolfram's Parzival*. New York: Oxford University Press, 2006.

Navran, Shakti Carola. *Jewelry and Gems for Self-Discovery: Choosing Gemstones that Delight the Eye and Strengthen the Soul*. Woodbury, Minn.: Llewellyn Publications, 2008.

Pelikan, Wilhelm. *The Secrets of Metals*. Translated by Charlotte Lebensart. Great Barrington, Mass.: Lindisfarne Books, 1973.

Prophet, Mark L., and Elizabeth Clare Prophet. *The Masters and Their Retreats.* Gardiner, Mont.: Summit University Press, 2003.

Randazzo, Sela Weidemann. *Rock-Medicine: Earth's Healing Stones from A to Z.* San Jose, Calif.: Blue Dolphin Publishing, 1998.

Raphaell, Katrina. *Crystal Enlightenment: The Transforming Properties of Crystals and Healing Stones.* Santa Fe, N.Mex.: Aurora Press, 1985.

———. *Crystal Healing: The Therapeutic Application of Crystals and Stones.* Santa Fe, N.Mex.: Aurora Press, 1987.

———. *Crystalline Illumination: The Way of the Five Bodies.* Kapa'a, Hawaii: Crystal Academy of Advanced Healing Arts, 2010.

———. *Crystalline Transmission: A Synthesis of Light.* Santa Fe., N.Mex.: Aurora Press, 1989.

Raulet, Sylvie, and Alain Boucheron. *Rock Crystal Treasures: From Antiquity to Today.* New York: Vendome Press, 1999.

Roeder, Dorothy. *Crystal Co-Creators.* Sedona, Ariz.: Light Technology Publishing, 1994.

Searight, Sarah. *Lapis Lazuli: In Pursuit of a Celestial Stone.* London: East and West Publishing, 2010.

Serrano, Ana Silvia. *Obsidiana: Piedra Sagrada de Sanación.* Mexico D.F.: Ediciones Indigo, 2006.

Silver, Dawn. *Jewels of the Lotus: Tibetan Gemstone Oracle.* Woodside, Calif.: Bluestar Communications, 1998.

Simmons, Robert. *Stones of the New Consciousness: Healing, Awakening and Co-creating with Crystals, Minerals and Gems.* East Montpelier, Vt.: Heaven and Earth Publishing, 2009.

———, and Naisha Ahsian. *The Book of Stones: Who They Are and What They Teach.* East Montpelier, Vt.: Heaven and Earth Publishing, 2007.

———, and Kathy Warner. *Moldavite: Starborn Stone of Transformation.* Marshfield, Vt.: Heaven and Earth Publishing, 1988.

Sperling, Renate. *The Essence of Gemstones.* Woodside, Calif.: Bluestar Communications, 1995.

Tag, Karin. *Das geheimnis der Atlantischen Kristall Bibliothek.* Hanau, Germany: Amra Verlag, 2013.

Temple, Robert. *The Crystal Sun: Rediscovering a Lost Technology of the Ancient World.* London: Century, 2000.

Trask, Mary. *The 12 Gemstones of Revelation: Unlocking the Significance of the Gemstone Phenomenon*. Shippensburg, Pa.: Destiny Image Publishers, 2009.

Twintreess, Marilyn and Tohmas. *Stones Alive! A Reference Guide to Stones for the New Millennium*. Silver City, N.Mex.: Ahhmuse, 1999.

———. *Stones Alive! 2: Listening More Deeply to the Gifts of the Earth*. Silver City, N.Mex.: Ahhhmuse, 2005.

Walker, Barbara G. *The Book of Sacred Stones: Fact and Fallacy in the Crystal World*. San Francisco: HarperSanFrancisco, 1989.

Warren, Thomas, and Sterling Gleason. *Ultraviolet Light and Fluorescent Minerals: Understanding, Collecting and Displaying Fluorescent Minerals*. Upland, Calif.: Gem Guides Book Co., 1999.

Williamson, Marianne. *A Return to Love: Reflections on the Principles of a Course in Miracles*. New York: HarperCollins, 1992.

Wright, Ruth V., and Robert L. Chadbourne. *Gems and Minerals of the Bible: The Lore and Mystery of the Minerals and Jewels of Scripture, from Adamant to Zircon*. New Canaan, Conn.: Keats Publishing, 1988.

Yamaguchi, Tadao. *Light on the Origins of Reiki: A Handbook for Practicing the Original Reiki of Usui and Hayashi*. Twin Lakes, Wis.: Lotus Press, 2007.

Zara, Louis. *Jade*. [n.p.]: iUniverse.com, 2001.

INDEX

BOOKS OF RELATED INTEREST

Stone Medicine
A Chinese Medical Guide to Healing with Gems and Minerals
by Leslie J. Franks, LMT

The Metaphysical Book of Gems and Crystals
by Florence Mégemont

Himalayan Salt Crystal Lamps
For Healing, Harmony, and Purification
by Clémence Lefèvre

Healing Stones for the Vital Organs
83 Crystals with Traditional Chinese Medicine
by Michael Gienger and Wolfgang Maier

Shungite
Protection, Healing, and Detoxification
by Regina Martino

Hot Stone and Gem Massage
by Dagmar Fleck and Liane Jochum

Power Crystals
Spiritual and Magical Practices, Crystal Skulls, and Alien Technology
John DeSalvo, Ph.D.

Vibrational Medicine
The #1 Handbook of Subtle-Energy Therapies
by Richard Gerber, M.D.

INNER TRADITIONS • BEAR & COMPANY
P.O. Box 388
Rochester, VT 05767
1-800-246-8648
www.InnerTraditions.com

Or contact your local bookseller